DEEP WALKING

A New Pathway to Health for Body and Mind

R. J. HOBSON

ISBN 10: 1483961923
ISBN 13: 9781483961927

For My Grandchildren:

Logan, Colter, Max, Caelan,
Hannah, and Benjamin

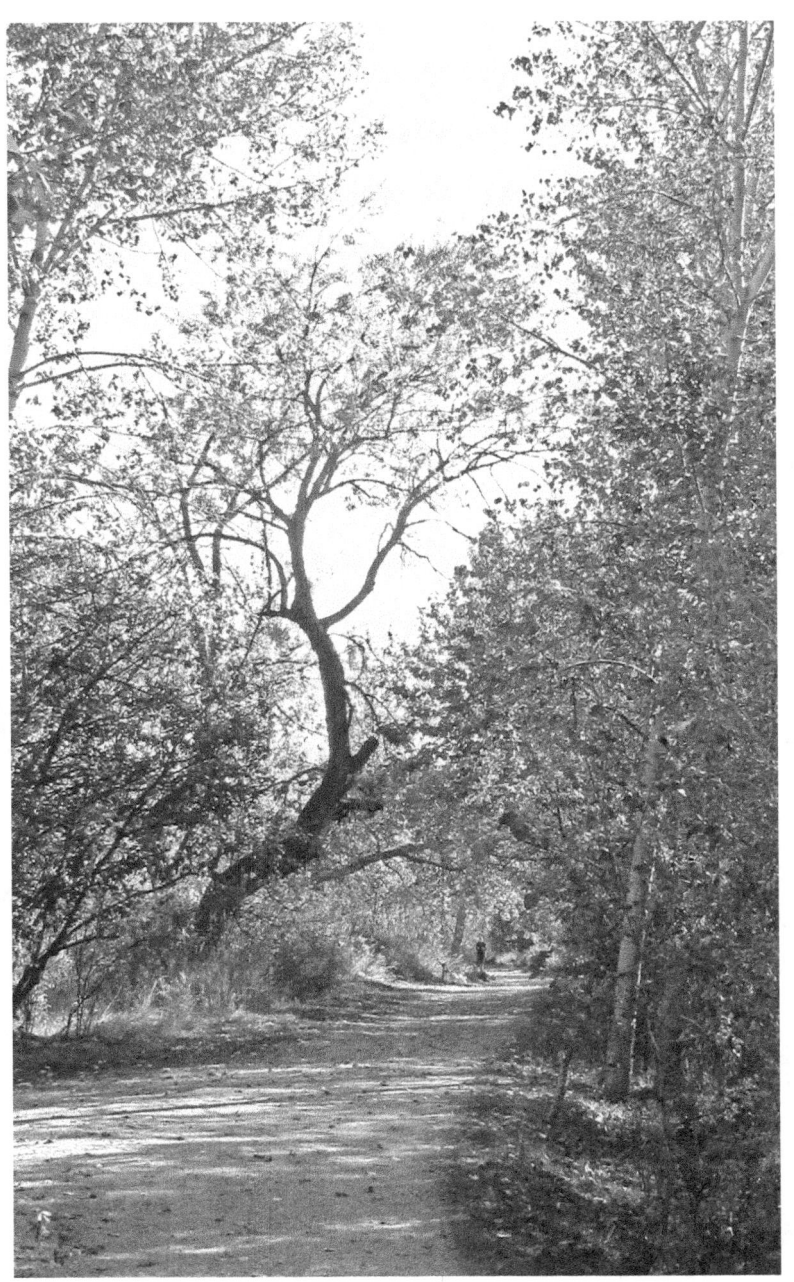

"Walking is man's best medicine."

— Hippocrates

"I have two doctors, my left leg and my right."

— G. M. Trevelyan

TABLE OF CONTENTS

PART 1

WALKING THE BODY

CHAPTER 1

INTRODUCTION

Hello, welcome to the walking path. Each word you read from this point forward will be like a single step which takes you closer to a healthier life. Word by word, step by step, we will progress to a new understanding of the importance of establishing consistent bodily movement into our lives and the cost to us if we fail to do so.

I am one of the "baby boomer" generation and I was born a few years after the Second World War, a horrific war where another generation risked and sometimes sacrificed their lives, and where millions of other heroic people made-up of innocent men, women, and children, were senselessly slaughtered. While the war was never a direct threat to my life, I am in my own way a survivor of that period in history, for a few years after the Great War ended I was diagnosed with a congenital heart defect and within my chest a child's small heart beat, but grew dangerously larger every day. Over time my enlarging heart increased to a size where it threatened to end my life soon after it had begun, so at six years old I was taken to Children's Hospital in Los Angeles for one of the first open-heart surgeries in the world. The doctors told my parents that I had a 50/50 chance of surviving the procedure, and of the three kids who had similar operations at the same time, I was the only one fortunate enough to survive.

As a survivor, I learned early in life just how fragile life is and I have never since my life-saving surgery taken it for granted. I consider it a gift to be able to participate in the walk of life, a gift I nearly lost when I was young, a gift many of us fail to fully appreciate because we have never come close to losing it. This year is the 60th anniversary of my heart surgery and my heart is still pumping, but I have learned that to keep it working properly I have to exercise routinely. While I had been physically active for most of my life, as I grew older I started to realize that I had been slowly decreasing my activity level. It was then that I began to read books and articles about walking and about the changes in our culture which have led to poorer diets and increased inactivity and which together now threaten the health and longevity of each of us.

After piecing together a walking regimen based on what I had read and fine-tuning that regimen for a few years, I decided to write a book about what I learned and to share that book with others. After all, I have received so much myself, from the doctors who saved my life, from my parents who got me help when I needed it and nursed me back to health, and from those who through their writings taught me about the current threats to my life and the best ways to avoid them. Now, I would like to pass some of this information on to you, and I hope it will change your life for the better in the same way it's changed mine. With that in mind let's begin.

First of all you should know that this book could save your life, and if it does not save your life it will at least extend your life and increase its quality to a degree beyond your ability at this point to imagine it. It will show you the way to decrease your chance of getting a terminal disease, help you lose weight and improve your self-image, and give you a generally greater sense of well-being by improving your mental health at the same time. I promise a lot don't I? I know I do, but as you will see the problem we may encounter is not the veracity of my offer or of my willingness to give it as a gift to you, but your reluctance to accept it and make it a part of your daily life. I know that too seems incredible, incredible that I should offer you the endowment of a higher quality prolonged life and that still you might refuse it. You might ask yourself, "Why would I refuse something like that, I am not a fool?" Please, let me explain.

The fundamental reason you might refuse my offer is rather simple. It's found in Newton's First Law of Motion which reads in part, "A body at rest tends to remain at rest unless acted upon by an outside force…" In other words, to accept my offer and receive your gift you will need to move your body more than you currently do, for if you are not moving your body enough it may take some outside force to help you do so. This book is an attempt to be that force, but please, if you would help just a little and not drag your feet. I will make it as easy as I can for you by providing the reasons you should start moving more and the consequences you will face if you don't, but in the end <u>you</u> will have to raise your body up, lean forward until you start to fall then catch yourself by moving your feet forward, beginning the process we know as walking.

So how can I suggest that something as simple as walking will improve the quality of your life and even prolong or save your life? It is because medical studies now show unequivocally that physical inactivity itself can speed up the rate of your aging, promote mental ill-health and contribute to numerous major physical illnesses and diseases. A direct correlation has been found between a sedentary lifestyle and increased levels of anxiety, cardiovascular disease, increased rates of mortality, deep vein thrombosis, depression, diabetes, colon and breast cancer, high blood pressure, obesity, osteoporosis, lipid disorders, sexual dysfunction, and even kidney stones. In general, inactivity weakens the immune system and depresses the natural healing capabilities of the body. Our bodies were designed to move and to operate optimally by being active. The problem is we are no longer as physically active as we were designed to be and the consequence is the deterioration of our health and erosion of our personal happiness.

Think about it. What would happen if we took a finely tuned race car that was meant to be driven daily at a high rate of speed and we only drove it once in a while at a slow rate of speed in stop and go driving? The answer is that the car would fall apart. By simply not using it often enough and failing to use it as it was meant to be used, our highly tuned race car would end as a heap of rust and sludge. It's the same with the human body; much of what we think of as normal aging is in fact unnecessary deterioration and decay caused by failing to use our bodies as they were intended to be used.

In their book, *Younger Next Year*, Chris Crowley and Henry Lodge, MD, state their belief that it is inactivity and not aging which is the primary cause of a life filled with illness, fatigue, and depression. It is not a natural decline of a well-oiled body machine which has worn-out due to normal wear but a decline we choose for it due to improper maintenance and by not using it correctly. We are literally decreasing the length and quality of or lives and wearing down not because we have been too active and suffer from standard wear and tear, but because we have not been active enough. Crowley and Lodge say that there is no reason that we can't feel as if we are age 50 well into our 80's, and that 70% of what we have come to think of as normal aging is optional, something which we choose.

When I started to go out for regular walks a few years ago and began to read some books and articles on walking, I learned a great deal about the serious consequences of physical inactivity. I was surprised to find that the science and research on these topics could not be more clear, inactivity is the new life stealer, and yet that fact is slow in arriving to the awareness of the general public. In fact few of the walking books I read provided readers with a sufficient amount of information about the deadly effects of inactivity and the relatively easy ways we might avoid them. Neither did they emphasize enough to my satisfaction the dangers inherent in our increasingly sedentary society. Let's take a moment to look at some of that information now.

According to statistics from the World Health Organization inactivity is the number one threat to public health in the 21st Century. Over 3 million deaths throughout the world each year are directly attributable to it, and millions more die each year due to illnesses exacerbated by inactivity. Add the two together and approximately 6 million people around the world die each year either due directly to inactivity or due in part because of it; it's a true world tragedy which could easily be avoided. Six million people, every year. If this number of people were to lose their lives annually for any other reason be it genocide, war, starvation, or disease, there would be universal outcry and international efforts to save those at risk. But in the face of six million deaths per year caused by inactivity, the world remains strangely silent. What is it that we read in the headlines of today which is more important than the preventable loss of six million people a year from the number one health threat of the 21st century? Where are the headlines about this? I don't know about the community in which you live, but in the one where I reside a front page headline about a world-wide epidemic of deaths caused by inactivity has yet to be seen.

The World Health Organization goes on to say that 60 to 85 % of people living in both economically developed and underdeveloped nations live sedentary lifestyles, and a sedentary lifestyle increases all causes of mortality, doubling the risk of cardiovascular disease, diabetes, and obesity, and all of the problems associated with these illnesses. The lack of physical movement for our bodies has taken over the role of being the number one cause of premature death in the United States and in the majority of countries around the globe.

Much of our sedentary lifestyle is one we choose because we select work which requires little movement and pick forms of entertainment which require little physical effort. I do understand that more and more jobs require long periods of time sitting and that in today's economy we take what jobs we can get. Still, while the solution may not be to find jobs that are more physically active, we can find other ways and times to move our bodies to the extent we should.

Another part of the reason we are more inactive than ever is because we feel the pressure of time and daily schedules and therefore select motorized ways to get around rather than walking or riding a bike. If people walked or rode their bikes everywhere they currently drive their cars there would be a dramatic health benefit to the general public. Many of us sit at work, sit while being entertained, and sit as we transport ourselves through our daily lives, and all this sitting is nothing short of deadly.

In the U.S. only 26% of adults engage in vigorous leisuretime activity. This includes actively participating in sports or working out three or more time per week. That means that 74% of us are not doing enough. As our amount of leisure-time increases our sedentary time increases also, and this is particularly true in the lives of our children. We all know the child "couch potato" phenomenon is a growing concern.

With the decrease of blue-collar jobs in our country and a shift to more jobs rooted in technology and the processing of information, we are less active at work and that is dramatically decreasing our level of physical activity. At work and at home we are moving less and sitting still for inordinate amounts of time as we stare at various screens. We are witnessing the cancer-like growth of something now called "screen time", daily time spent sitting with our eyes glued to screens large and small either as a requirement of work, an issue of convenience, or entertainment choice. With increased screen time, studies show that the American lifestyle is becoming more sedentary, and that lifestyle has become a silent epidemic pushing the statistics of childhood and adult obesity and premature mortality through the roof, robbing us not only of the quantity of years we have to live, but of the quality of our lives as well.

There is no doubt that all this inactivity contributes to the escalating number of people suffering from heart disease, diabetes, and cancer. The next time you attend a funeral, remember, while you can tell that the person in the casket is dead because they do not move, in ever-increasing numbers there is a good chance that the person is lying in a casket in the first place because they did not move enough while still alive. To express Newton's famous law in another way, "A body at rest which rests too much tends to move to a state of permanent rest."

The temptations to be inactive are great. Many of us who have sedentary jobs have little choice about our decreased body movement in that portion of our lives. The lure of television, video games, and social media is great as well and with the ever-increasing growth of our use of technology and increased screen time the future does not look bright for a return to a time when physical activity is the cornerstone of our work and play. So what to do? The answer is simple. We have no choice. While we can choose to be sedentary and to be fat rather than fit, we cannot choose whether the result of that choice leads to obesity, heart disease, cancers, and depression. It's a given. If we have a sedentary job and choose sedentary leisure-time, the choice is simple: make time for regular physical activity or accept the fact that you will have a shorter life filled with fatigue, illness, and loss.

If I were to ask you to list all the things that were more important than your health what would they be? If you are like most people the list would be very short. If I were then to ask you to make a list of the things you actually do on a daily basis to guarantee you maintain your health, what would that list look like? If you are like most of us there would be a glaring discrepancy between what you consider to be important for your health and what you actually do to promote it.

What is more important than your health? Most people respond to that question by saying that there is nothing more important than their health for without good health there is no quality of life, and without good life quality there is really nothing at all. It is almost a cliché, "You have nothing, if you don't have your health." Yet again when people are asked what they do each day to ensure good health the answer is slow in coming. We all know that without good health we lose the quality of our lives, and in worst case scenarios lose our lives completely, and in social settings when the subject of health arises we can all talk eloquently about the importance of health and the need for good nutrition and exercise. Still, in many cases, when it comes right down to doing it, there is a disconnect between what we say and what we do. Perhaps at last it is time that we make the switch from lip service to leg service, and not just be someone who is talking the talk of good health, but becoming someone who is actually walking the talk.

CHAPTER 2

ACTIVE OR INACTIVE?

Today we are learning more and more about the increasing level of human inactivity around the globe and its effect on people everywhere. The already long list of preventable mental and physical health problems grows longer every year. As we have seen, our lack of physical activity is one of the leading causes of preventable death throughout the world, and our growing sedentary lifestyles and lack of exercise can contribute to or be a risk factor for a variety of illnesses and diseases. Still, as I researched the information which is easily available concerning our poor diets and growing inactivity levels, I was not prepared for the amount of incontrovertible evidence showing that humans on this planet have taken a new a dangerous path toward collective ill-health. It is as if we are all traveling in a large car together, a car we call the modern world, and that car has just turned a corner and we now see in our lane up ahead a semi truck speeding directly toward us. This is not hyperbole. The threat is real, but the truth is that the threat is not coming at us from outside like a runaway eighteen wheeler but is actually riding inside the car with us. The threat is in fact largely created by we ourselves, by poor choices in diet and activity levels which are hurling us headlong into an inevitable and deadly collision. Throughout this book I will provide you with just a small sampling of the statistics and research which reveals the frightening truth about our possible future. I do so in the hope that after reading them you will do as I did, look for yourself at some of the current studies and research on these topics then quickly reach for your walking shoes.

According to the American Heart Association, cardiovascular disease is the leading killer of women over age 25. It kills nearly twice as many women in the United States than all types of cancer, including breast cancer. Only 13 % of women think heart disease is a threat to their health. Nearly one third of U.S. adults have high blood pressure, and high blood pressure is a major risk factor for heart disease, stroke, congestive heart failure and kidney disease. According to the Center for Disease Control high blood pressure is listed as a primary or contributing cause of death for over 350,000 Americans each year with the numbers continuing to grow.

In many cases, increased levels of heart disease is related to our societies' dramatic gain in weight. Almost two-thirds of U.S. adults age 20 or older are overweight, about 62% of women, and 71% of men. Nearly one-third of American adults are so overweight they are considered obese with less than one-third of all American adults age 20 or older maintaining a healthy weight.

The primary reason for the rising numbers of over-weight people and cardiovascular disease can be traced to our changing lifestyles. Again, we have become more and more sedentary and remain inactive for most of the day with little or no exercise. This lack of exercise causes muscle atrophy, the shrinking and weakening of muscles which can lead to a susceptibility to physical injury. Because fitness is related closely to immune system function, reduction in our fitness level is generally followed by a weakening of the immune system as well, directly affecting our ability to fight off disease. A review in *Nature Reviews Cardiology* suggests that a sedentary lifestyle can also negatively impact natural elements of the healing process like inflammation which can become non-adaptive in unfit individuals and lead to the development of chronic illness. In other words, our inactive lifestyles are not only increasing our susceptibility to illness, they are making us ill, and making it much more difficult to fight off illness once it strikes.

What other factors contribute to our being inactive? Besides the fact that we are involved in less physical activity in our leisure time and jobs and our domestic lives have become more sedentary as we use passive modes of transport, environmental factors contribute as well. It is difficult to exercise in environments where there is violence, heavy traffic, poor air quality and pollution, or in the growing number of neighborhoods which lack recreation centers, or in some instances lack parks and sidewalks.

In times past, exercise and other body strengthening activities were the way we often spent our leisure time. We recreated at parks with baseball diamonds, basketball courts, tennis courts, playground equipment and open spaces in which to run. But now as a society we have turned inward and not in terms of introspection, but turned inward into our homes where we sit in front of various screens to either virtually socialize or wait passively to be entertained. The only thing increasing as fast as our national weight average, blood pressure levels, and new diabetes cases is our screen time. Much of the time we call leisure time is spent in front of the television set and much of our work and school time is spent in front of screens as well.

Of the sixteen hours a day in which most of us are awake, the average American now spends one fourth of that time watching television. That's one fourth of our waking lives staring at the tube. Add to that the amount of time we spend at home or on the job or in school sitting in front of a computer, and the time we spend with those miniature screens on our hand-held devices, and you will realize that many people spend one half to two thirds of their lives sitting around and staring into flickering screens of various size. Think of the toll this takes on our bodies, the bodies that have evolved with a need to stay moving, and which actually require movement to be healthy. If movement and action is what our bodies require to live, no wonder we are aging and dying faster than we need to, and why our increasingly resting bodies are inclined to stay at rest.

In the 2008 United States American National Health Interview Survey, 36% of adults were considered to be essentially sedentary and 59% of adult respondents never participated in vigorous physical activity lasting more than 10 minutes per week. The *British Journal of Sports Medicine* says that those of us who watch six hours of television a day shorten their lives by an average of five years, while those who exercise just fifteen minutes a day add an average of three years to their lives. The statistics are endless, but all begin to signify one sad fact: our inactivity is killing us. How many times have we heard this cliché line in a movie,

"I think he is dead."

"How do you know?"

"He isn't moving."

Well, when it comes to our quicker-paced health decline and aging do to inactivity our characters might say:

"I think he is going to die very soon."

"How do you know?"

"He isn't moving as much as he should."

Fortunately there is a corollary to Newton's law that a body at rest tends to stay at rest, and that is that a body in motion tends to stay in motion. In the world of physical activity that translates into: a body that moves continues to move, or simply, a body that exercises is healthier and lives longer. The antidote for all of the maladies precipitated by inactivity is a daily regimen of movement. In fact the answer to all of the following questions is exactly the same answer, and not perhaps the answer one might expect.

How do you control your weight? With fad diets and exercise gimmicks? No, you do so through regular body movement. How do you decrease your risk for cardiovascular disease? With blood pressure medicine? No, through regular movement. How do you reduce your risk for Type 2 diabetes and metabolic syndrome? With strict diets and continuous insulin injections? No, through regular movement. How do you reduce your risk for some cancers, for weakened bones and muscles? Through movement. How do you improve your mental health and mood? How do you improve your ability to do routine activities and prevent falls if you are an older adult? How do you increase your chances of living longer?

Again the answer is the same for each: through consistent daily body movement.

So now we know some of the horrific consequences of inactivity for both our current health and future health, and know too that movement is the key which can open the door to a brighter future and to a more fulfilling life right now. If you are inspired to move by the information you have just received then you might ask, which type of movement should I choose? Aerobics, Yoga, Pilates, tennis, health clubs, golf ?

While these are all fine options for the diverse tastes and interests of individuals, I recommend something much more basic, something we were all born to do, in fact something we have done most of our lives and a natural movement built into our essential selves. I recommend walking. We were literally born to walk, and I would suggest that by once again walking at the levels we were designed to walk we all might be, in a sense, reborn.

Walking for humans is as natural as breathing and, like breathing, sustains us. It is a movement that can be done by everyone, people of both genders, people of all races and ethnicities, and by people of all ages. And the good news is that moderate-intensity aerobic activity, like brisk walking, is generally safe for most people. With a good pair of walking shoes, a commitment to 30 minute walks several days per week, we can transform our current life and brighten the outlook for our future. It might seem like a big promise for such a small commitment to such a simple activity, but I assure you, after a few months of regular walking you will find a little extra spring in your step, be smiling more often, look forward to the next opportunity to walk, and wish you had discovered the magic of increasing your amount of walking time many years before.

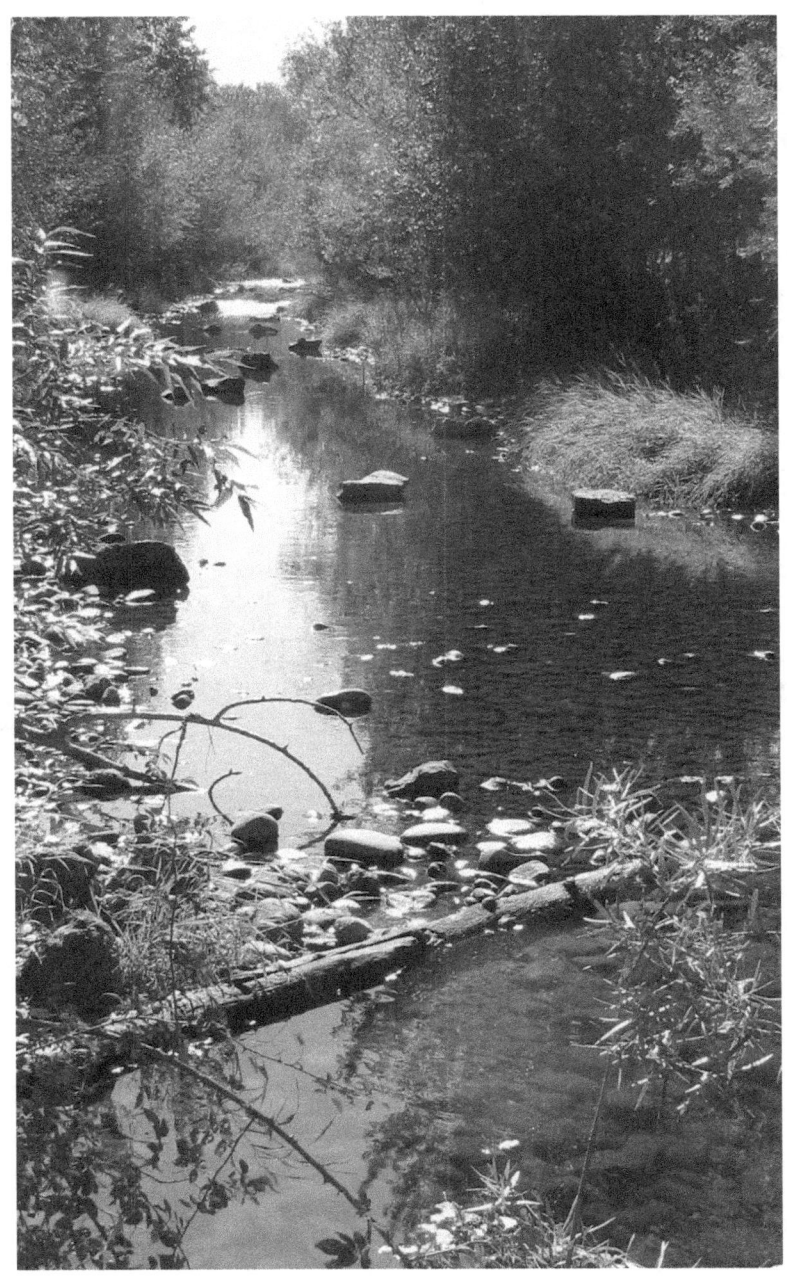

CHAPTER 3

WHY WALKING?

I suggest that you begin a lifelong walking routine for a variety of reasons. Here are a few of them. First of all walking is a popular exercise, in fact studies show it to be the most popular exercise. Part of the reason for its popularity is that it is easy to do, requires no monthly expenditure for a gym membership, no great investment in specialized equipment, and can be done by a majority of people by simply walking out their front door. It is also easy to do while traveling and can be done to get from one place to another, what is known as "active transport," unlike passive transport, such as driving a car to all of our destinations. Walking is a low impact activity which causes minimal stress and injury to the body and is an action which comes to us naturally and promotes health to all of the natural systems of the body. But is it really exercise? The answer is definitely yes, and the benefits are immense.

While not as rigorous as some workouts, walking nonetheless has fantastic benefits and helps to assuage the many symptoms of aging as well as combat many human illnesses and diseases. According to the Mayo Clinic, research shows that regular brisk walking can reduce the rate of heart attack the same amount as a more rigorous exercise, like jogging. In fact one study showed that men who jogged less than one mile per day had twice the mortality level of men who walked two miles every day. And women's cardiovascular systems benefit from walking as well. In the Nurse's Health Study (72,488 female nurses) those who walked three hours or more a week reduced their rate of heart attacks and other coronary events by 35% compared to women who did not walk.

Walking also helps in the prevention of Type 2 diabetes. The Diabetes Prevention Program has shown that walking 150 minutes per week and losing just 7% of our body weight (12-15lbs.) can reduce our risk of diabetes by 58%. In fact, getting out and walking for 30 minutes a day is a minimum daily requirement to help prevent Type 2 diabetes. A study by the Graduate School of Public Health, University of Pittsburgh, discovered that walking for 30 minutes a day cut diabetes risks for overweight as well as non-overweight men and women, and walking also helps maintain blood sugar balance for those with diabetes.

Walking is also good for our brains. Like other exercise, walking leads to the release of the body's natural feel-good chemicals: endorphins. After walking, most people notice an improvement in mood, and a 1999 study published in the Annals of Behavioral Medicine showed that university students who walked and did other easy to moderate exercise regularly had lower stress levels than inactive people or even those who exercised strenuously. It has been found that walking also helps alleviate symptoms of depression. Walking for 30 minutes, three to five times per week for 12 weeks reduced symptoms of depression as measured with a standard questionnaire about depression and its numerous deleterious effects by an amazing 47%. Not only does walking have a positive effect on one's general mood and help reduce anxiety and depression, it can actually help cognitive function. Researchers found that women who walked 1.5 hours a week had better cognitive function and less cognitive decline than women who walked less than 40 minutes a week. A study of people over 60 funded by the National Council on Aging, published in the July 29, 1999 issue of Nature, found that walking 45 minutes a day at 16-minute mile pace increased the thinking skills of people over 60. The participants started with 15 minutes of walking and built up their time and speed, resulting in the participants becoming mentally sharper after taking up this walking program. Here are some other important benefits to walking.

Walking everyday promotes weight loss. If we move at a brisk pace we can burn 240 to 440 calories per hour of walking. This adds up and we can shed a pound or more per week and that adds up to 52 lbs per year. In fact, if we simply add just 2000 more steps a day to our regular activities, we may never gain another pound. Research from Dr. James O. Hill of the Center for Human Nutrition at the University of Colorado Health Sciences Center suggests not only this but argues that adding in more step exercise such as walking is an important part of any weight loss program. Of course, we must still watch what we eat and how much we eat in order to lose weight, but walking helps build healthy lean muscle, burns off inches of fat, and increases metabolism. Successful weight losers, and those who keep it off almost always maintain a program of walking or some other routine exercise.

One of the first things we notice after we begin a walking regimen is an increased energy level. Increased movement seems to actually not tire a person but invigorates them. For some this is counter intuitive, thinking that more activity will make a person feel more tired. But the opposite seems to be true. Perhaps it is one of the reasons, "A body in motion tends to stay in motion."

Walking everyday will also help us feel good about ourselves. Self-esteem is bolstered when we do something which benefits us and as we start to feel and look younger. The mental changes and transformations brought about by a simple regular walking routine are astounding. Others will begin to notice often before we do. They will quickly see the physiological changes and the effect walking has on our overall sense of well-being, and note that we just seem "happier."

Walking is also very good for our bones. Research shows that postmenopausal women who get out and walk approximately one mile each day have higher whole-body bone density than women who walk shorter distances, and walking is also effective in slowing the rate of bone loss from the legs. We know also that walking provides greater lubrication to the joints and helps to promote joint healing and dramatically slows the effects of joint deterioration. Some research even shows that walking reduces the risk of breast and colon cancer. Women who performed the equivalent of one hour and fifteen minutes to two and a half hours per week of brisk walking had an 18% decreased risk of breast cancer compared to inactive women. Many studies have shown that exercise can help prevent colon cancer and even if an individual develops colon cancer, the benefits of exercise appear to continue, both by increasing quality of life and reducing mortality. Not only does walking and exercise reduce our risk for breast and colon cancer, it is also good for those undergoing cancer treatment, improving their chances of recovery and survival. For men, walking regularly has even been shown to help prevent erectile dysfunction and reduce the risk of impotence.

The truth is, walking generally improves all physical function. Studies show that it not only improves fitness but prevents physical disability in older people. We know that it promotes healing in the ill and infirm and stimulates the immune system which helps keep life-shortening diseases at bay. We know that walkers live longer. The Honolulu Heart Study of 8000 men found that walking just two miles a day cut the risk of premature death almost in half. Other studies have had similar findings, and it is difficult to deny that if we keep walking consistently we improve our chances for a longer and healthier life.

As you can see, we really asked the wrong question at the beginning of this chapter. The question is not "Why walking?" The question is really, "Why have we not been walking more all of our lives?" Again walking is a natural and needed body activity nearly as crucial to our health as drawing air into our lungs. Would we consider breathing less or quitting completely? Of course not. Like stopping or curtailing our breathing, when we slow down and stop moving at healthy levels we slowly begin to die at an ever increasing pace. But on a positive note, when we start getting back to healthy levels of movement we begin to increase longevity, and improve the quality of the longer lives we have to live.

CHAPTER 4

HERE, LET ME GET THOSE EXCUSES FOR YOU

After hearing the consequences of increased levels of inactivity and the incredible benefits of regular walking we might think that a gift like increased health would be easy to give away and be even easier to receive. The What's the Most Important Thing in Your Life question I mentioned earlier with its nearly unanimous popular response, "health," might make us think that people would receive an offer of better health unequivocally. But while people are receptive to the gift of health they are often unwilling to receive it once the understand that it requires time and effort on their part. Once they learn that they will need to actually make time to walk and expend a little energy, the ideal of increased health and happiness seems far less important than it did initially. To be given something that requires no work is one thing but a gift that requires work and a change in lifestyle however small is different.

Our very own ingrained cultural value of seeking the easiest way to do things contributes to the problem of inactivity, and is also in part responsible for the difficulty we experience when trying to break the inactivity cycle. Because we are inclined to seek the easy way, the way which requires little or no work when trying to accomplish a task, we often resist doing any additional work to that which we are required to do. While the easiest and most convenient way might work successfully in some life situations: convenience stores for quick shopping, instant breakfasts to save time, pills to lower blood pressure, it is unsuccessful when it comes to increasing the daily amount of time we move our bodies. There is no other way to move but to move; there is no shortcut, no instant fix, no pill. And unfortunately no one can increase our activity for us. In this case the buck stops here, with each of us, you and I.

So how does one reconcile the contradiction between stating that health is our number one priority and a failure to actively do something about it? Why is it easy to see this hypocrisy in others and fail to see it in ourselves? We do so by seeing ourselves as different, special, the exception. "Everyone really should go to the effort; they are really crazy if they do not, but its different for me. You see, I have my reasons, extenuating circumstances." It is here with the belief in personal exceptionalism that the panoply of excuses begin, and it becomes like that cliché metaphor for the arguments going on inside our own heads where an angel sits on one shoulder and a little devil sits on the other. The angel knows that we would benefit greatly from increased exercise and is all for it, but the little fellow on our other shoulder provides a barrage of excuses as to why it's not for us. We need to pay very close attention to what this dark little cynic is telling us. Perhaps as you have read this book he has spoken up already? If so, what are his excuses? As we explore the top 10 excuses people use to avoid exercise, lets see if our own little inner naysayers are at least original in the excuses they create.

In his book, *Deep Medicine,* Dr. William Stewart, cofounder and medical director of the Institute for Health and Healing at the Pacific Medical Center in San Francisco states the following: "Everything you think, feel, say, and do is either health creating or health negating. Everything." This is a truly insightful and amazing statement with far-reaching implications. While it is easy to see how choices in activity level and diet have consequences to our health, it is more difficult to see the subtle ways that our thinking has consequences for our well-being. In this book we will discuss in detail the relation of physical activity to mental health in later chapters, but at this point we need to understand that our ability to think clearly about becoming more active may already be distorted by our lives of inactivity. Just like our bodies, if they have been mostly at rest, balk at increasing their movement, (A body at rest tends to remain at rest) the mind too becomes sedentary and creates excuses and justifications for the body not moving more.

Before we get started we must acknowledge that there are real reasons why someone cannot increase the level of movement in their lives, physical limitations being the most obvious one. But I am going to assume that if you have purchased a book on walking, that you can walk. And I am going to conclude also that if you have picked up a book on walking, you realize you need to do something more than you are currently doing to promote your personal health. The little angel on your shoulder has gotten you this far, so let's work together to defuse the negativity and excuse making the little fellow on your other shoulder may already be whispering in your ear. So he won't have to exert himself by stretching and contorting to make excuses, so he won't have to move his weary bones mustering up rationalizations, so he won't have to make any effort to live longer, enjoy greater energy, and avoid illness…here, let's get those excuses for him. Here now are the Top 10 excuses people give for why they don't engage in regular exercise; they range from the 10th most popular to the most popular excuse of all.

10. **I Don't Enjoy It** ----- If this is one of the excuses that comes to mind perhaps we need to redefine what the word joy means to us. Maybe we are confusing the word joy with the words pleasurable, comfortable, and easy. Once we understand the benefits of walking and realize we could have more of life to live and an increased feeling of well-being and optimism how could anything but joy be the final result? If we cannot enjoy better health and happiness what can we enjoy? Many inactive people begin to associate happiness and joy with laziness and inactivity. "It's better not having to do anything isn't it?" This thinking is in fact a form of mental laziness which often comes with a sedentary lifestyle. It is "object at rest" thinking and a form of rationalization which justifies inactivity. It is obvious that someone who does not move much would not find joy in moving, just as someone used to moving would not find joy in sitting on their backsides most of the time. The "I Don't Enjoy It" excuse is not a reason not to move more through walking, it is a symptom of the inactivity disease already at work within us. We need to start to see this excuse for what it is: an indication of just how ill we have become and our need to learn how to find joy in being active. If we change the way we define joy we will change our lives, and have a far better quality of life to live.

9. **I Don't Want To Be In Pain** ----- No one wants to be in pain. For that reason in the chapters ahead I recommend very slow and cautious levels of increase in the development of our more active lifestyle. On the other hand we need to make a distinction between pain and discomfort, and recognize that a little discomfort is really the complaint of a rusty machine asked to work again, complete with plenty of squealing and squeaking. Discomfort is not a sign we are doing something hurtful to ourselves but a sign of just how far we have let ourselves go. We must start to see any slight discomfort we feel as a sign that we are getting healthy and breaking the crippling effects of being sedentary, of sitting and being still, and their ultimate consequence: being dead. Discomfort is our liberator. Remember, the discomfort we feel as we begin to be more active will decrease over time as we get into better shape. Remember also that whatever discomforts we feel in the beginning phases of exercise pale in the face of the discomfort and pain of obesity, low self-esteem, or coronary bi-pass surgery.

8. **I Am Not Fit Enough** ----- Not fit enough? If we are not fit enough to slip on our walking shoes and step out the door then we have a problem of a serious medical nature. Putting on our shoes, dressing ourselves, and stepping out into the world is the minimum physical requirement for beginning a walking regimen. Again, let me emphasize, if we cannot meet this requirement we have a problem which is serious enough to warrant medical attention. However, if we can do those things and do not have any serious current medical problems we are fit enough to walk. If we can put on clothes and step outside and just take one step then turn around and go back inside we are ready, and on the next day we can step

outside and take two steps before returning to the house. Do that, and we have begun a long and beautiful journey. With every step our fitness level will increase giving us the ability to take additional steps after that. The old expression coined by Chinese philosopher Lao-tzu, "A journey of a thousand miles begins with a single step" could not be more suitable than when applied to the beginning of a new life achieved through walking. And the benefit of that journey does not come somewhere near the end of our new-life walking routine, but in the heart of each and every day we walk.

7. I Am Not Motivated ----- A lack of motivation to do something comes from simply not believing it is important enough to do. Perhaps you do not like to run, but if a tiger were chasing you you might be surprised at how quickly you change your mind. You would see a sudden and dramatic increase in your interest in running and your willingness to do so. If it helps just think of ill-health and premature death as the tiger on your heels. If we are not motivated after reading the information in this book and under-standing that a choice not to walk or to do some form of exercise is ultimately a choice to age and die prematurely and accept a life of illness and suffering then chances are nothing is going to motivate us. If we do not have the will to live, or lack concern about having optimal health there is little that can be done.

For me, a lack of motivation to do something which improves and prolongs my health which is relatively simple to do is a no-brainer, particularly if we value life and all that it contains. What-ever one's theology or philosophy of life might be, it seems obvious to me that life is a sacred gift which is bestowed upon those of us who are currently living. For me, to take this gift and dishonor it by not caring for ourselves is the ultimate insult to the gift giver and to one's self. I can understand how ignorance, not knowing the facts about health and aging and the consequences of inactivity on our lives might leave us unmotivated to get up and move. But once we know the truth, how can we continue living as we have? Don't we see that light in the eyes of our friends and family, our children and grandchildren? Aren't we curious about life's next chapter, what will happen to all of those we love and who love us? Each day that I go for a walk I think about how fortunate I am to be able to walk, and I think of that old aphorism, "Those who can walk, should walk." For me it is not only about valuing the gift and being around to share life with my loved ones, it is about the quality of my life, the one I live each day, the quality of my energy level, and the level of my daily joy.

Not long ago I bought three little Hotwheels monster trucks and gave one to my five-year-old grandson Max and one to his little brother four-year-old Colter. I kept the other for myself. We played on the floor for what seemed like a short time but which turned out to be an hour, scooting around the carpet which we pretended was a terrain made up of hills, rivers, and canyons where our Hotwheels trucks drove endlessly. When at last I got up off my hands and knees I realized I still had my pedometer on, the one I wore when I started my own walking regimen. When I looked at it I saw that I had traveled well over a mile in the last hour. A mile, scooting about on my hands and knees crawling happily around with my grandchildren. When I told my daughter, the boy's mom, she laughed out loud while the boys encouraged me to rejoin them back on the floor, "Come on Pops, let's go. Hurry up." Soon I was back on the floor. For a brief moment I did not think about playing with monster trucks but about the joy of living and the wisdom of my choice to stay active, and to overcome the excuses of lethargy and the lack of motivation which ultimately comes from a lack of gratitude for the opportunity to live. "Come on Pops, let's go." I say the same to all of you. "Come on, let's go."

6. **I Have No Energy** ----- **Any** low energy levels we become aware of in the beginning of an increased activity regimen are the result of our past lifestyle. It will take a little time to change. After all, movement makes it easier to move just as sedentariness makes it easier to sit. Low energy is not an excuse not to exercise, it is a reason to exercise. We should think of our low energy levels as a warning signal, a warning that we have started slipping away from good health, for low energy levels generally only get lower. Low energy is nature's way of telling us that we are not active enough. If a person has developed over the years a lifestyle of decreased movement, the feeling of having no energy is inevitable. Changing that energy level will take time, but it will change, for once people start moving more the result over time is renewed energy. We may have also created some poor eating habits which match our poor exercise habits. With increased exercise these too will often change. When we begin to feel better and more energized we will find we may want to begin to eat better also. Our healthier bodies will demand it. We shouldn't be at all surprised when consistent exercise starts changing our metabolism, increasing our energy levels and producing endorphins, improving our mood and thereby stimulating our body energy and mental vigor and optimism as well. And at the same time, our new positive self-esteem kicks in and our spirits rise as we desire more and more to be active.

Low energy levels when we are currently inactive or have been inactive in the past are as much mental as physical. Part of the reason that "a body in motion tends to stay in motion," is that our mindset after exercising for a time begins to shift. Before long the message in our brain will begin to change from "I have no energy," to "what am I going to do with all this extra energy?" So remember, the lack of energy we may feel initially is a trick our sedentary selves are playing on us to keep us sitting down and the consequences of having already sat down long enough. We can't listen to the lazy trickster inside our heads, but simply move ahead, and in a very short time we will be surprised to feel a new level of energy growing within us.

5. **I Don't Know How** ----- This might at first sound like a silly complaint, particularly since we are talking about walking. And while we all know how to walk, the truth is that walking has a few complexities and subtleties we might not think of even though walking is for we humans a very simple thing to do. This book will discuss the nuances of beginning a walking regimen not everyone might think of as well as present information about the specific benefits of doing so. While we certainly know how to put one foot in front of another in order to move forward, this book will provide us with the knowledge we need to have in the areas not so obvious. We may not "know how" to walk in all its forms and subtleties but soon we will, and the excuse of "I don't know how" will fall by the wayside like all of the rest.

4. **I Have Children** ----- The last thing we can do is let our children be the excuse for the neglect of our wellness level and

general health. Our children and grandchildren if we have them should in fact be a major motivation for improving our health. If we cannot find a minimum of 15-30 minutes in the 16 hours of the day we are awake to be away from any children we need to care for then it is time not to give up but time to get creative. Perhaps a friend or family member, or a spouse or partner can watch any children for the short amount of time required for us to take a walk. Perhaps the kids can walk with us or be pushed in a stroller as we walk. Maybe we will have to get a treadmill and walk inside at home, or watch and move to an exercise tape instead of leaving home to take a walk. There are countless ways we can find to move under even the most limiting of lifestyles or parenting responsibilities.

To use our children to excuse ourselves from exercising when in fact we should be exercising so we can better care for our children and continue as a presence in their lives is disingenuous. If we put some regular exercise in our lives we will be a happier, more energetic parent for our children and a role model for developing kids who need to grow up understanding the importance of exercise. Perhaps then our children won't find themselves in the out-of-shape condition we now find ourselves in. Can't walk because we have children? Wake up, we need to be walking more because our children and grandchildren and others we love need us as healthy and happy influences in their lives.

3. **I Have a Specific Physical Injury** ----- It is amazing how those old bodily injuries from our past suddenly act up at the mere thought of more exercise. Often times we confuse normal stiffness and soreness with a real injury, and sometimes after a little exercise old injuries which never fully healed or incorrectly healed

will remind us that they are still there and need more work. If these injuries are not very painful we should begin walking very slowly and walk only a short distance. In other words, we need to adjust the speed at which we walk, and how often we walk in our walking routine so as not to overly stress the weak spots in our physiology. These weaknesses can range from a stiff ankle due to an old soccer injury to a more serious weakness in cardiovascular conditioning. There will be a list of conditions in next chapter on assessment which are serious enough to seek medical advise about before you start walking. So if it turns out our injury is serious enough to prevent us from walking at all, we will have to heal that injury first so that we can begin to heal our more serious injury, a body which is not receiving sufficient movement to maintain good health.

2. **I Can't Afford It** ----- This popular excuse for avoiding exercise has little value for those thinking about starting a walking routine. The costs of walking are minimal. Aside from comfortable shoes and clothing, and the pedometer I recommend, there is little investment needed for an activity which gives its practitioners such tremendous benefits. In fact walking could be called the least expensive exercise known to man and that is part of the reason it is also the most popular.

1. **I Have No Time** ----- Well here it is, the number one excuse used around the world to justify not making the effort to improve one's physical and mental health. Once examined, this excuse turns out to one of the flimsiest of all and the contrast between this claim and reality make it one of the most pathetic and humorous. "I have no time to take care of myself," is really the

claim, "I have no real interest in caring for myself and I will turn to laughable excuses to prove it." With a national average of 240 minutes per day of watching television, the suggestion that we cannot find 30 minutes a day to exercise is ludicrous. How can those of us who are awake for 16 hours per day, a total of 960 minutes, claim not to have 30 minutes a day to prolong our lives and make our lives more energized and free of illness and disease?

We all know the demands of time and lives which are generally hectic if not chaotic. It often feels like there is just not enough time in the day to get the things done we think we need to do. So just what are the things that are so important, more important than our health? Watching television certainly isn't one of them, and if we go through our daily list of activities one by one, and hold them up to 30 minutes of daily walking and the benefits it brings, the majority of our list will be exposed as trivial by comparison. Building a healthier life is a bit like creating a beautiful sculpture, but in this case we are both the artist and the work of art which we create. The magnificent marble statue forming in front of our eyes is our creation, the person we want to become, the chips and dust which fall away our impotent excuses. The "I have no time" excuse is really saying, "I would rather do something else, anything rather than exercise." And that more honest admission is one of two things: an ignorance of the consequences of failing to be physically active or an acceptance of our deteriorating health, something we see is as inevitable, a basic kind of giving up. Have no time? The object of this program is to give us <u>more</u> time, more time to truly enjoy our lives and to have more time to live.

Well, there we have the top 10 excuses not to increase our physical activity to benefit ourselves and improve our lives. I am sure that you will agree that once examined they are all pretty weak. How does anyone actually believe their own self-deluded excuse making? The answer is that they are excuses people tell themselves when they are in a weakened state, suffering from the stupefied inertia of non-movement, and people looking for any excuse to stay that way. It is a deadly combination, a person who is good at making excuses coupled with a willing listener who wants more than anything to believe them.

CHAPTER 5

ASSESSMENT

I hope that the preceding chapters and the information they contain about the consequences of inactivity and the benefits of regular exercise have motivated you to start a walking program. For me, once I learned that information the choice whether or not to increase my daily amount of movement became a critical life-altering decision and not just a choice of whether or not to add something "I should do" to an already busy life. I recognized it in fact as nothing less than a very clear choice between a good quality or poor quality life, between ill health or wellness, between joy or sadness, loss or gain, life or premature death.

By this time in your reading of this book you have probably already decided if adding regular walking to your life is important or not and if you are going to revitalize your life or retreat to the lifestyle you have lived in the past. For those of us who are ready to go forward into a life of greater health and happiness we must begin by assessing our current amount of daily body movement. That amount will serve as the baseline for understanding what needs to be done in order to elevate our conditioning activities and reveal our current fitness level.

Before beginning a walking regimen, it is a good idea to consult your physician. If any of the following apply to you it is not an option to consult one but a necessity to do so.

You have bone or joint problem such as arthritis.
You are breathless after limited physical exertion.
You have pain in your chest, neck, arms and shoulders after physical exertion.
You sometimes have dizzy spells or feel faint.
You have been told my a doctor that you have high blood pressure.
You are pregnant.
You smoke.
You have any other type of medical problem which might keep you from starting a walking program.

If none of these problems are holding you up then we can continue forward with our assessment of the current amount of movement in your life and determine what amount of additional movement is needed. It is important that this assessment be accurate. I recommend that you purchase a pedometer in order to make that assessment and to monitor your progress particularly in the beginning of your new walking regimen. Pedometers record our daily step count, an excellent indication of the true amount of movement we engage in during the day. They come in a wide variety of types and have varying features and prices which range from five dollars to a hundred dollars. You can pick them up at most sports shops and even many drugstore chains. The one I use cost about twenty dollars and attaches to the pants or shorts at the hip. It automatically resets itself at midnight, and keeps my step totals for several days in case I want to review them. I like to record my daily step count on a calendar like the one I describe at the back of this book just to get an idea about my daily average and to give me a visual display of my exercise consistency. Pedometers do not lie; they give us an objective record of our movement so we know when to do more or less to satisfy the goals we have set for ourselves. In my opinion increasing the amount of movement in our life without the use of a pedometer---at least initially--- is like trying to lose weight without scales. We need an objective indicator. So how many steps are enough?

The generally accepted standards for step count health is as follows: 5000 steps or less per day indicates a sedentary lifestyle, 5000-7500 steps is the current American adult average, 10,000 daily steps is the desired amount for optimal health needed for an adult based on health studies, and 12,500 or more steps a day is considered highly active. Remember, 2,000 steps equals approximately one mile.

What we then need to do is to determine our current average step level and then supplement it with a walk or a number of short walks which will get us over time to the 10,000 step level. Once we are consistently getting the daily recommended step count of 10,000 we will begin to see benefits from our walking in both our physical health and in our mental health.

Without the use of a pedometer, it is easy to fool ourselves into thinking that we are doing enough in our daily activities to get the exercise we need. We all think that we work hard, that we get as much movement as most people, and that we are generally active and not sedentary. It is not necessarily so. I recently read an article by tennis great Martina Navratilova. In it she talks about her first use of a pedometer after she retired from tennis. Although she had been retired for some time, she still believed that she lead an active life. True, she no longer practiced tennis daily or played in tournaments, but she worked around her home and cared for her beloved dogs, 16 of them. Each day she took them for a walk around the block, but because she had so many, she took them two or three at a time. It seemed to her like a lot of walking. She was shocked after wearing a pedometer the first day and discovering that her daily step average was about 7,800 steps, well below the 10,000 steps recommended for adults. She had assumed that the dog walking was keeping her fit, and it was helping, just not enough. I had a similar experience.

When I first purchased my pedometer, I wore it on my hip and went about what for me at that time was a normal day. I had been retired for a few years and lived alone so in the morning I went about doing my routine chores of bed-making, light house cleaning, laundry and such. I next went to the market to stock up on food supplies then went online to answer e-mails before going to meet with a family member later that afternoon. My evening hours were typical: making dinner, talking to family and friends on the phone, watching a little news on television, listening to music and reading. After preparing for bed I went to my calendar and prepared to write down my first step count ever. I saw on my pedometer that I had taken 5432 steps for the entire day. I was very surprised. From my point of view it had been a somewhat busy day and yet my pedometer indicated that I was only 432 steps above being sedentary.

When I had worked in the past my job was physically demanding and included a lot of walking and physical effort. I knew I wasn't getting the same amount of daily movement after I retired but that was to be expected; I was retired after all. My pedometer showed me just how much daily movement had been lost from my average day and the weight I was gaining indicated that I was beginning to pay a price for my decreased activity level while at the same time maintaining my regular eating habits. I knew I would have to supplement my step count each day with some form of consistent daily work-out. Somehow I needed to add nearly 5,000 steps to my day in order to get to the 10,000 steps recommended to stay sufficiently active. I realized not only that I had decreased my activity level dramatically since retirement but also that a person has little understanding of exactly how much they are moving without the aid of a pedometer. I had been staying busy after my retirement, but I learned that busy and getting the necessary body movement I needed to are two very different things. It was at this time that I supplemented my normal movement during the day with a period reserved for daily walking.

After we determine our daily step count average the next thing to do is to figure out what time of day is easiest for us to go for a walk. This in part will be determined by whether or not we are able to walk directly from our home or if we will need to travel in order to get to a walking path. Security is also a factor to consider (more on this later) as is whether or not we will be walking alone or with a pet or other person. Most importantly of course we will have to consider our daily schedule. Will we be able to walk at the same time each day we walk, and if so when? Ideally I believe it is best to walk at nearly the same time each day so we can establish a routine. If we have a specific time each day set aside for our walk we will be more likely to walk regularly than if we try to work a walk into our daily activities when it is convenient. Our walk must become a priority with most of the other activities of our day being adjusted to fit around our walking time rather than the other way around. If, as most of us believe, health is our most important priority, then prioritizing it over other things is the logical thing to do. A good friend of mine calls his daily walk "the foundation of his day." We wouldn't build a house without a foundation would we? Only when we too begin to think of walking as our foundation will we make sure it happens regardless of what other things are on our daily "to-do" lists.

I have found that for me an early morning walk works best. If one's walk becomes the foundation of the day then like a house foundation there is an advantage to building it first; it keeps our house from falling down. I have found that an early walk sets the tone for my entire day because I have started my day with time for myself, and begun my day with an activity that will help insure that there will be many good days to come. It was from that routine walking time which was set aside in the morning to affirm my life through positive physical effort that the rest of my day was built. I then built on that first day of the week's physical activity the next day then each day after that until I had constructed a week of consistent walking. From that week of walking I constructed a month of walking and before I knew it the months added up to a year of consistent walking. After a year I realized that by walking one morning at a time I had built a new life which had as its foundation a simple consistent life-affirming routine demonstrating my belief in myself and my love for the life I was living. Now I think of walking as building the foundation of my life one concrete block at a time, and the more blocks one has in their foundation the stronger it becomes.

At one level it matters very little if you walk in the morning, afternoon, or evening, little at least compared to the fact that you are walking on a regular basis. While I enjoy starting my day with a walk, a walk in any other part of the day is satisfying as well, so if you can't walk each morning, walk in which ever part of the day you can, but try to do so consistently.

How we begin our walking regimen is important. Not just the light stretching I recommend in an upcoming chapter before we walk, but the way in which we take our first few walks. The object is to start walking gradually, gradually as in slowly, gradually as in for shorter lengths of time in the beginning. Think of the first few walks themselves as important warm-ups. If a person has been relatively inactive, or has not been walking for any length of time on a regular basis, they should begin walking in a way which will not overly tire them or create discomforts which might be discouraging. We want this experience to be pleasant, relaxing, and satisfying. We can push ourselves more later, after we have toned up, but not in the beginning. In the beginning we want to end our walks feeling like we want to do more, not less. This way we will look forward to the next day when we can go out again, not to be dreading it because we are stiff and sore. In other words, we want to be good to ourselves. We are easy on ourselves in the beginning understanding that this is the beginning and that in the natural progression of our new walking lifestyle we will eventually walk faster and further. Be patient.

Our use of a pedometer is extremely important when starting a new walking regimen. Later, once we determine how much we need to add to our daily level of movement with regular walking throughout our week, and begin to do so, our pedometers are less important. We will eventually develop a sense of how long and far we need to walk each day based on the other activities we have planned and our knowledge of approximately how many steps they contribute to our daily step count. Still, I like to wear a pedometer every once in a while just to make sure I am not unknowingly slipping away from the amount of steps I know I need and make any adjustments necessary.

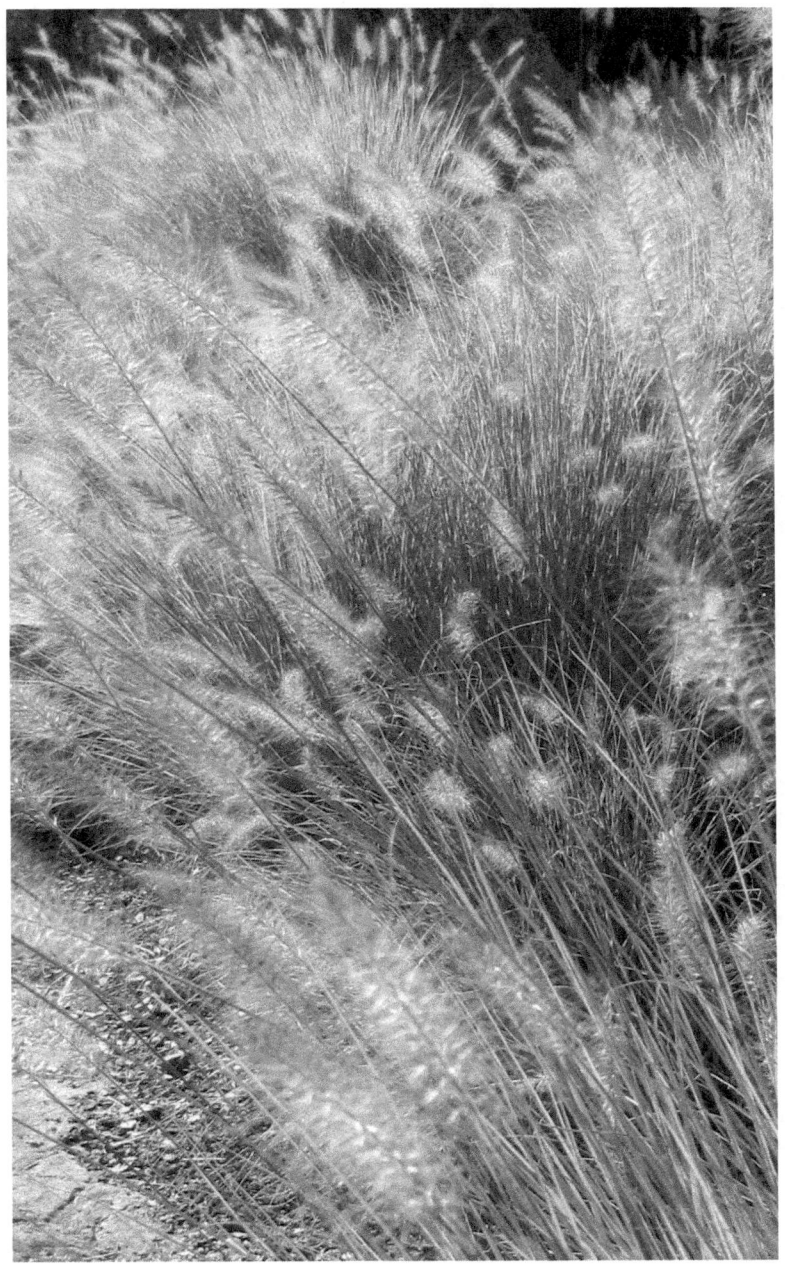

CHAPTER 6

SETTING REALISTIC GOALS

Why have goals? The answer is that many of us like to know that
the efforts we make will lead to the consequences we desire. However, having completely inflexible goals leads to some very serious
problems: disappointment and discouragement when we fall short
of a goal, built in limitations of how far we can go with rigid goals,
and the fact that rigid goals can create a counterproductive emphasis on goal-based motivation. In the first instance if we set a goal
of say losing ten pounds of weight in two months and in fact we
lose six pounds we can shift from a once positive attitude about
getting out and walking each day to a less optimistic one. In the
walking regimen suggested in this book attitude is everything. I
want participants to leave the house feeling optimistic and coming back feeling even more so. There are enough negative "you-
are-less-than" and "you-don't-measure-up" messages in our culture
without bringing them into our walking space, a space we want to
keep supportive, encouraging, and affirming. Still, seeing progress
in some form is beneficial. So how can we have both, goals to assist

progress and yet goals which don't give us false motivation or suggest the possibility of failure?

I believe we need to have flexible goals, goals which are not hard and fast and to which individuals must conform but rather goals which flow around each person's efforts to a degree yet continue to lead them forward. To do this we must keep our goals generalized. For example, such a goal might be to make progress over time with weight loss without attaching a specific number to that goal. Or we might keep a record (as described in Appendix 1) of our feelings as our energy levels increase without quantifying them with specific numbers and other labels which suggest that some numbers are good and others bad and that some represent success while others represent failure. In cases where we are trying to achieve a hard number goal, like completing 10,000 steps per day, we can still see it as a goal we are working toward but do not see a day of less than 10,000 steps as a letdown. We must always remember where we started from, and recognize that even our smallest number of walking steps in a day is better than the time when we took very few or no walking steps at all.

Every single step has value, for it is a step toward better health and increased happiness. We need to keep in mind that numbers are neither good or bad or indicative of success or failure; they are simply reference points by which to judge our progress over time. Another reason I am against setting rigid goals is that rigid goals will not keep us walking, and that is really our primary goal in both the beginning and the long-term. If we need fixed goals to keep us motivated what do we do when our goal is achieved? Set some higher goal? When we achieve 10,000 steps a day do we shoot for 20,000? When we lose thirty pounds do we work to lose fifty pounds? Where does it all end? A ninety pound skeleton walking endlessly around the neighborhood?

While I hope we will stay away from developing rigid goal-based thinking in our walking program because it leads to a form of black and white, success or failure thinking, I also hope we learn that we do not need the achievement of distant ideals to feel successful. Goal-minded thinking often leads to the perception that success lies in the future with a person we have yet to become rather than focusing on the person we are now and the success we enjoy each day. One thing walking teaches us is that the present moment is already something wonderful and the person we are now is wonderful as well. Walking helps to center us in the moment and free us from the idea that all good things exist in the future and that the rewards of our walking regimen will be found there rather than existing each moment as we put one foot in front of the other and celebrate each moment we are alive.

In our walking program we will keep only one eye casually looking toward the future. Any long term goals will be soft goals, general milestones to encourage us and to make us feel successful when we accomplish them. In the beginning our goals will be very subjective and flexible focusing on how we are feeling, how our thinking is changing, and on all the other positive changes going on inside of us. We are concerned mostly about now, for if we act and think in a healthy way today and every day, the future will take care of itself.

The essence of all choices and other creative acts lies in the present moment, not in some time before now or after now. In the creative act the past helps us very little, and in fact can hold us back because it creates an expectation based on what we have done before and encourages us to use ideas and methods we have already used rather than developing new ones. What good does it do us to remember that we have never succeeded at keeping weight off in the past or that we have started exercising before but did not keep it up? And the future truly does take care of itself for it is really nothing more than the resulting sum of all of our current choices, and that is why the formation of the new self which we desire will begin and end in the moment. It is the reason too we emphasize our current state of mind as we walk and as we prepare to walk, and how we think of our walk once it has been completed. Mindset, again, is everything, and that mindset operates now, in the eternal present, and that is where our work is done and our new life unfolds.

Many of us see walking as a metaphor for living. Think of Dire Strait's Mark Knopfler and his song "The Walk of Life." That is why we often see the dynamics of the daily walk as much the same as those of our life walk. The old model we have lived where we let our current potential be defined by past performance and allowed some dream of the future be the carrot which moved us forward is bankrupt. We must replace it with the new model which is centered in the now. And we can use that new model not only in our daily walking but in all aspects of our lives. The truth is that many of the problems we now face and are trying to overcome, ill health, excessive weight, depression, habitual behavior and addictions, are the result of living in the old paradigm where the past defines us and we wish for a future where we are somehow magically improved. Both of these strategies make us feel inadequate now. Change this way of thinking and we will change our essential self. The walking program described in this book will help us do just that, and for that reason when we talk of setting goals we mean setting goals for each day rather than setting goals we hope to realize in the future. I would rather see a smile on our faces as we put an "x" on our calendar for having walked another day and enjoyed a beautiful walk then see a frown develop on our faces as we stand on the scales and focus on our failure to reach a desired weight in a desired period of time. Our future is now and we should not forget it.

CHAPTER 7

WALKING GEAR

One of the great advantages of having walking as our primary exercise is that it is relatively inexpensive. No club memberships are necessary, no green fees, elaborate rackets, skis, or clubs. If walking is the poor man's exercise it may be part of the reason that people with less money are slimmer than those with lots of money. Yes, it could be an issue of food quality and quantity as well. Still, cultures where walking is commonplace due to economic necessity have a populace which weighs less and who enjoy greater fitness than those whose inhabitants use motorized vehicles to go everywhere. I like to think of walking as the people's exercise, an activity as old as mankind itself and a common gift which we all share. The problem again is that the majority of us just don't do the amount of walking we were designed to do.

Shoes, specifically walking shoes, are our most essential acquisition, and it is very important to be selective and to try them on before we buy them. This may seem obvious, but I have known those who have ordered walking shoes out of catalogues or online and that is definitely not the way to go. We need to buy our shoes where we can try them on. Here are some things to look for.

First, we need to be sure the heels on our walking shoes are low and slightly rounded in the back or are even slightly beveled. As we walk our feet roll forward from heel to toe and it is important that the heel does not impede this movement. A thick heel or heel which flares out can make a correct walking motion difficult and even slow us down or cause shin and knee discomfort.

Because our feet roll from back to front as we walk it is important to make sure that the soles of our shoes are flexible. Try bending and twisting the shoe's sole. Compare it to a running shoe which is usually much stiffer.

The upper section of the shoe needs to be light and made of material which breathes. The last thing we want is a heavy shoe made from leather which cannot bend or breathe. We want the feeling that we are treading lightly over the ground not clunking along in hob-nailed boots.

Obviously of primary importance is making sure that our shoes fit properly. Our heel should not lift up when we walk and we should have room for our toes to move. We want about one half of an inch of space between our toes and the front of the shoe and wide enough so our toes can move freely side to side yet with minimal space. When our shoes are laced up and we walk in them we should not feel that they are pinching us either across the top of our foot, over the ball of our feet, or anywhere around our toes.

People's feet tend to swell a little later in the day, particularly if we have been on our feet a lot. Go looking for shoes in the later rather than in the early hours of the day; we want to fit our shoes when our feet are at their largest not their smallest. We also need to take our walking socks to the store with us so we can see how our new shoes will fit while wearing them, and we need to make sure to try on both shoes as they can vary slightly in size as may our feet.

When shopping for walking shoes it is important to take time to shop carefully. We can't run in and grab the first stylish shoes we see and which seem to fit well enough. Remember, this is our most important walking purchase, literally where the rubber meets the road, and if we can get a more comfortable pair of shoes with a better fit for a few dollars extra we should not hesitate to do so.

With our receipt in hand we need to return home and wear our shoes around the house for a time before we venture outside with them. Wearing them for an extended period of time is the only way to really make sure that they fit and by not taking them outside they will be in better condition if we decide we need to return them. They should be returned if while walking in them we feel any discomfort, if they bind anywhere when we walk, our heel rises up, or any "hotspots" develop on our feet. Most stores will allow the return of and exchange of shoes if they are not damaged.

In the Appendix on record keeping we will discuss the importance of keeping a record of our walking outings. One thing we will keep track of will be the number of steps and miles walked both on a daily basis and over time. The reason for doing this is not only to keep a record of our accomplishment but to keep track of the number of miles we have put on our shoes. At 300-600 miles not only will we be fit beyond our most optimistic hopes but our shoes will be wearing out, losing their ability to support our feet sufficiently. My hope is that we will all wear-out numerous pairs of walking shoes. If our shoes are very light weight, if we are over-weight or wear our walking shoes at times other than walking for exercise we will wear out our shoes faster and have to replace them closer to 300 miles than to 600.

Other than shoes, all we will really need for walking will be the pedometer I have recommended already, and the clothing you will walk in. The clothing needed obviously depends on where one lives and the time of year we are walking. If you are like me and live in an area where there are four complete seasons, I would recommend the layering approach to dress and wear clothing that does not absorb perspiration but wicks it away from the body. If you are in a colder and wetter climate or have such weather during part of the year then you will need a fleece layer as well as a layer of waterproof covering.

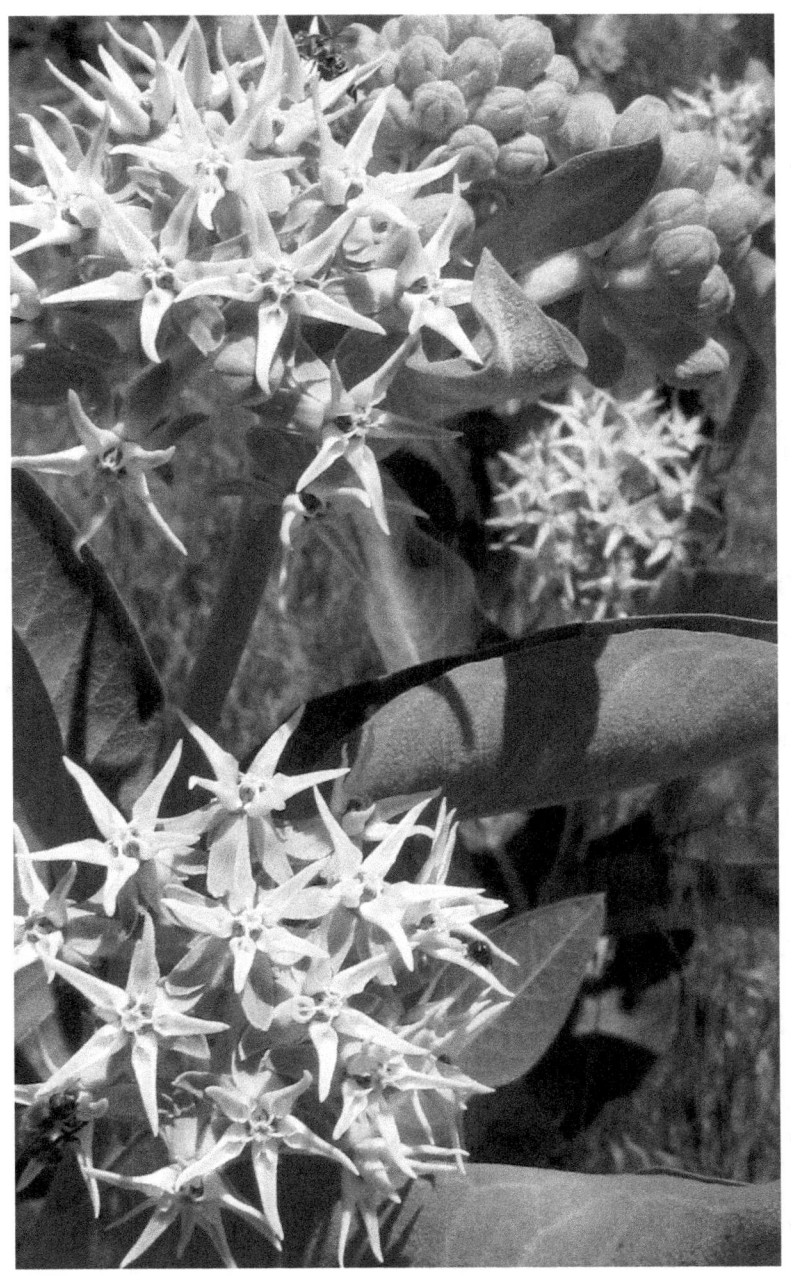

CHAPTER 8

TREADMILLS

While I have a prejudice in favor or walking outdoors and in a natural setting whenever possible, sometimes that is difficult to do. If we have other options which include using a treadmill either in our home or gym then I recommend using them when we can't get outdoors due to inclement weather or any other problems. Our number one priority is to walk and to walk on a consistent basis. In other words, we want to walk anywhere anytime in anyway we can. If bad weather prohibits walking outdoors, walk indoors. If there are small children who cannot be left alone in our home, we walk in our homes rather than putting off walking until a time when we can get free. If we have a rigid work schedule and need a quick and easy walk and have access to a treadmill then by all means we should use it. Treadmills may not be as nice as walking in nature and getting out of the house, but they are a wonderful alternative to not walking at all.

When I first began walking I would walk twice daily. I would get up early and be on my walking path no later than 7 a.m. then walk again in the late afternoon. The problem was that it was summer time and it was incredibly lovely out in the early morning hours, a condition unfortunately not consistent throughout the year where I live. During that first year I stuck with this walking schedule through the early and middle Fall, until it starting continuing to be dark at 7 a.m. and frost started to appear and eventually there was snow. At first I started waiting to go on my walk until later in the morning to have more light and warmth but over time my morning walk began to intrude into the time for my afternoon walk, or at least into the recovery time I needed between my two walks. Finally I gave up my morning walk and walked only in the warmth of the afternoon sun. It didn't take long for me to realize that I was decreasing the number of my daily step count and when full-blown winter hit on some days I had difficulty getting out at all. It was then that I purchased a treadmill for my home.

I admit that I was cynical about treadmills initially, seeing them as providing an "unnatural" exercise compared to my usual exhilarating walks in nature. I found myself wishing that I was outdoors instead of stuck inside, in an artificial environment, walking on a man-made machine. Over time however I started to enjoy some aspects of this type of walking. Sure, I missed the fresh air, the natural sounds and smells, and beautiful sights which surrounded me outdoors, but soon I began to discover that walking on a treadmill was not the totally inferior way to get daily movement into my life I thought it was. In fact it provided some unique opportunities and different perspectives on the whole walking experience.

There was no doubt that using a treadmill had the convenience factor going for it. It was easy to lace-up my shoes and step into my exercise room and before I knew it my morning walk was done. But that was not the main appeal. I also liked the fact that I could regulate and keep track of my walking speed better, for I had to walk at a consistent pace or risk falling off my treadmill. I was also able to regulate the degree of incline which gave me as intense a workout as I desired. To get this option in my outdoor walking, I had to choose from varied walking routes all over town and get myself to them. I would eventually learn that my indoor winter walks with their varied speeds, durations, and inclines would aid my conditioning and improve my walking skills when I returned to walk in the natural settings I preferred in the Spring. In short, my treadmill helped me get into better condition faster and easier then I could when taking my usual walk outside.

Where I was truly surprised by my treadmill walks and training sessions was in the area of mental health training. My treadmill turned out to be a natural meditation machine. There were fewer distractions competing for my mind's attention, and I could control my surrounding indoor environment making it easier to control my mental focus. I began to explore different in-house environmental settings. I could make the room very quiet with the exception of the rhythmic sound of my feet striking the surface of the treadmill. I could even close the drapes and darken the entire room except of a small light which shown on the treadmill's surface so I would not lose my balance in the dark. The deprivation of the visual sense and the limiting of sound to an almost drum-like beat as my feet hit the treadmill's rotating belt helped me to gain control of my thoughts and enter into an almost trance-like state. The truth is that by using the treadmill to abstract and distil my walking experience, it made it easier to for me to enter the mental states I desired to enter and which I can now more easily enter when I walk outside in nature.

In summary, I soon found that my treadmill benefited not only my physical conditioning by making it easier for me to create more challenging walking workouts, but it also helped train me to enter very relaxed and healing states my mind. In future chapters I will discuss the importance of trying to achieve these mind states which are used in our over-all effort to use walking to heal and condition both body and mind.

It should be noted also that the new generation of treadmills that now exist contribute other features which make indoor walking more interesting and fun. While my treadmill is not one of the more expensive varieties, it still has some unique features. These include speakers and Mp3 player capabilities. I can have music if I want it or listen to books created in an Mp3 format, and language tapes as well. It even has a built-in fan which helps keep me cool when I need it. The most interesting feature my treadmill has is its capacity to link with the internet. There, I go to a website called Ifit where I can create walking routes using Google Maps. Once I create a walking route, I can see that route on the screen of my treadmill. From Paris, France to Paris, Texas I can walk on my treadmill and actually see the route I am walking either from an overhead map-view, close-in satellite view, or in Google's amazing "streetview". In "steetview" as I look at the screen on my treadmill I see every detail of the area I am walking in as if I were walking down the street, and as I walk on my treadmill it appears that I am proceeding down the street. I have walked the streets of Paris and London, trails which run beside the ocean on the west coast, through the red rocks of Sedona, Arizona and numerous other beautiful places throughout the U.S and around the world. As I walk, my treadmill adjusts its incline to fit the terrain I am walking over, making it possible for me to determine where I walk, at what speed I walk, and how much up-hill terrain there is depending where I choose to walk. My walks can range from easy to difficult and I can save any maps I make for myself online. On occasion before traveling to unfamiliar cities I have walked them on my treadmill, and it has made getting around those cities much easier. I remember once in Amsterdam telling the cabbie the easiest way to get to my hotel. He asked if I was a local or had spent time in Amsterdam in the past. I explained to him that the only time I had been to Amsterdam was once before, in my exercise room back home in the U.S.A.

Again, I have a definite prejudice in favor of walking outdoors. More and more, we live in an artificial world and I believe that in many ways that self-selected artificiality injures our physical and mental health and dehumanizes us all a little more each day. Nature is our element. It heals and restores us, and re-centers our very being. We must always keep in mind that our goal in walking is to heal our illnesses and restore our health. To allow that natural process to proceed we must put more nature in our lives, more natural foods, more natural movement, more natural settings, and a more natural pace of life. Still, I believe that it is important to have as many varieties of walking options available as possible to make sure we walk consistently and to give us the variety we need to keep us interested and thereby keep us walking. I would therefore recommend that our walking on a treadmill remains our second best option but an option nonetheless.

CHAPTER 9

PERSONAL SAFETY

Obviously it is important to be safe while walking. If we are indoors on a treadmill, no problem. However, if we are walking outdoors we need to be more cautious. The precautions we take for personal safety completely depend on if there are in fact any threats to our safety in the places that we walk and what those threats are. You will be the best judge about your safety because you know best what your local safety issues are, where you will be walking, and the condition of your own health. If we are new to an area, or even if not, we need to be sure we do a little research and talk to those who are already walking where we will be walking and get the advice of our local safety agencies as well. While there is no such thing as being able to walk with absolute safety, or for being able to get out of bed each day for that matter, the odds of our being safe can be greatly enhanced if we use some common sense guidelines. First we must identify the types of safety concerns there are. Threats come from a wide variety of sources: people, animals, automobiles, trail hazards, and possibly even our own lack of physical conditioning.

Safety threats from people

The best way to defend ourselves from possible threats to our welfare from others is to either walk where there are always people around whom we feel safe with or to always walk with a walking buddy be they human or canine. The larger ones are more intimidating. That applies to both human walking companions and dogs. Some walkers carry pepper spray, sound alarms and even electric shocking devises. I would suggest that rather than walking in fear which is very detrimental to the relaxed mind states we want to attain, that we go with a friend or spouse, or join a walking club. I would even prefer that one uses a treadmill or walk inside the local mall rather than turning something as beautiful and liberating as walking in a natural environment into a time of constant concern, nervousness, and fear. We are doing this after all to heal ourselves, not to generate more sickness.

Safety threats from animals

Once again, you will be the one who knows best whether animals are a threat to you where you walk. There are mountain lions on some walking trails in California; there are numerous moose and bears in walking areas in Alaska, but for most of us off-leash aggressive dogs are the biggest threat. Most owners are good about controlling their dogs, but on occasion we may run into a dog walking without its owner. If so, it is important to remain cool, and if the dog is not blocking our way continue on. The worst thing we can do is freak out. We just stay calm, don't make aggressive movements toward the dog and relax. If there is no other option we turn and walk back in the direction from which we have come. Where I often walk I have gotten to know both the people I see routinely on

70

my walks and their dogs as well. Even those who were at first wary of me now come up and lick my extended hand. I am referring to the dogs now and not the people.

Automobiles

Many of us do not have the opportunity to walk in car-free areas. Those of us who do are blessed. For those of you who have to be near automobiles as you walk be sure to make yourself as visible as possible. Wear bright colors including safety vests and other such clothing. Do not plug your ears with music devices; we need to hear everything around us. Obviously even when walking near traffic we should stay as far from it as physically possible, and choose routes with less traffic when possible.

Trail Hazards

When I speak of trail hazards I am not thinking of something like people on bikes although in some areas they would qualify. I am speaking of hazards we find <u>on</u> the trail, things like potential stumbling hazards which can either be on the trail or be a part of the trail. When we are focused on our walking, or just lost in thought about other things it does not take much to trip us up. First of all, we should try to find a walking trail with few trail hazards or if we know the trail has hazards pay closer attention to where we place our feet. This will come naturally once we pick ourselves up off the ground a time or two. I admit I enjoy the road less traveled, the path less taken, a trail less walked by others and which provides a little challenge in incline or takes me into places of greater natural beauty. The kind of trail where one has less of a chance being passed by a jogger than a deer. We shouldn't avoid these areas if we are safe in all other ways; we just need to be extra careful. Actually, careful and concerted focus on our foot placement as we walk can help us enter into a wonderful "in-the-zone" type of mental state that is extremely relaxing and healing. We call it mindful walking. More on this later.

Poor conditioning

Our own conditioning or lack there of can well be our greatest safety concern. Once again you and your physician are the best judges in this regard. If there is even the remotest possibility that we could have a health issue while walking due to some preexisting condition, we should not walk alone. At the very least we carry a cell-phone which is not bad advice for all of us as long as they are not constantly ringing and disrupting the pleasure of our walk. If we do have a health problem for which we might suddenly need assistance, it is best for us to continue walking with others or where others are walking nearby until our conditioning improves in both our opinion and that of our doctor's. We can work toward the goal of walking alone if you like that idea, but once again, we must use common sense. I repeat, we should not under any circumstances put ourselves in a position where it is difficult for us to get help if a health condition we know we have can put us at risk. It is not worth taking the chance.

A few other walking safety tips

We need to avoid walking at night alone or where there is poor visibility. If we walk at dawn, dusk or into the early night hours we should wear reflective gear. We also want to know our walking trail or route well, and do not just head out, destination unknown, and should make sure someone else is aware of the areas we routinely walk in and the general times we go there. If you are a woman do not dress seductively, and men and women should not wear visible jewelry. Again, it is generally best not to wear headphones at all, but if you like listening to music as you walk plug your player into only one ear. The bottom line is not to call attention to yourself, and to be as aware of your surroundings as possible.

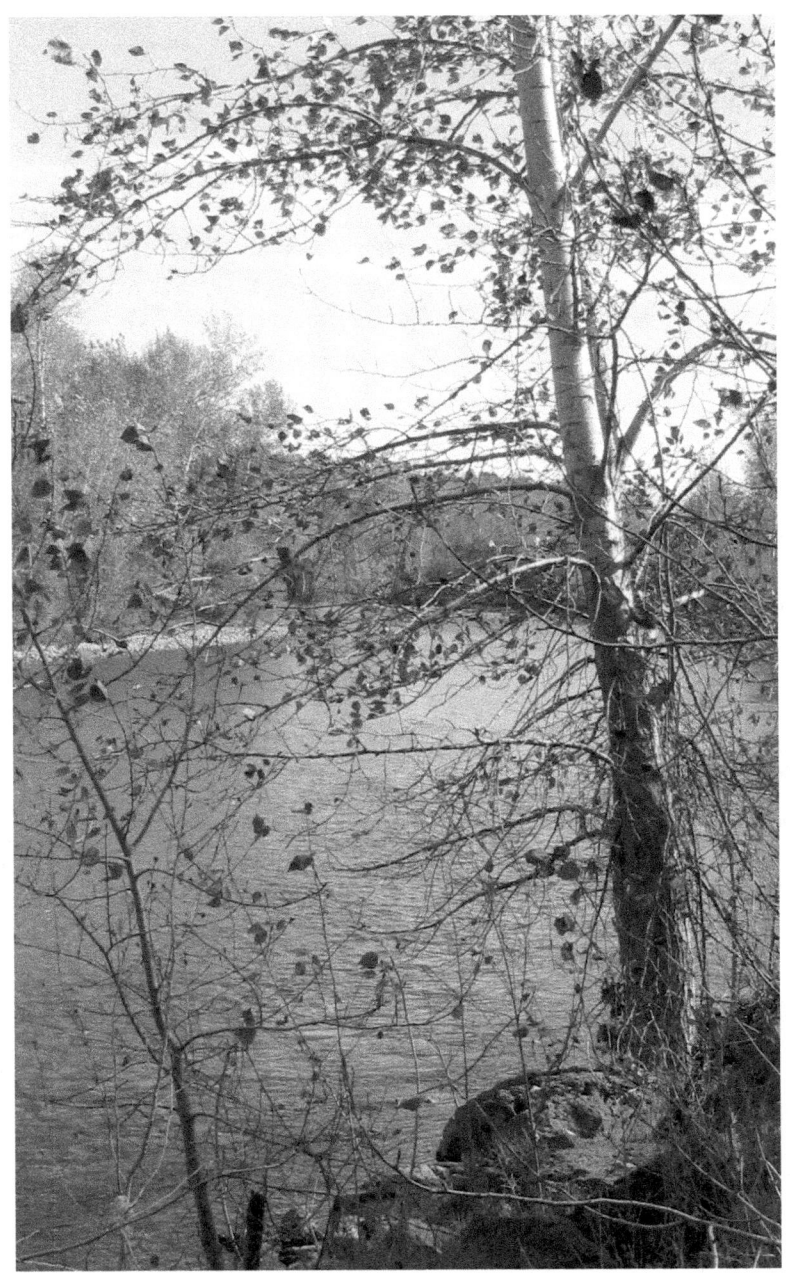

CHAPTER 10

SOLITARY WARRIOR OR TRIBAL MEMBER

The decision of whether to walk by ourselves, with others, or with a pet is each of ours to make, but here are some things to consider. First of all we may have no choice; we may have a pet or friend or mate who is extremely passionate about walking with us. In that case often the decision is made for us, at least for some of our walks. If not, or if we are excited about going out on our own, we are choosing to be primarily solitary walkers and that can have some very real benefits. The reason that people walk with pets or other people is usually either because they want security and companionship or feel obligated in some way to do so. While these reasons are often good ones for having a pet or others with us, there are other things to consider.

To get the full benefits of this walking regimen I would suggest that at times we walk alone if security is not a factor. If security is a serious factor I think it is important enough that we walk alone on occasion that I suggest that we find a spot where we can safely walk on our own at least from time to time. Why?

In future chapters in which we will discuss the mental benefits of walking we will see that one of the great perks of getting out and doing something beneficial for ourselves is that it helps to create a sense of personal empowerment. Many of us have spent much of our lives working on behalf of others or continually living or working in tandem with others. And sometimes we have been other-based to an extent that we have neglected ourselves, or at least failed to show ourselves that we value ourselves enough to make time just for us. Changing that habit is one of the central benefits this walking program has to offer. I want each person who follows this plan to develop a deep and abiding respect and caring instinct for themselves based on, in part, their personal effort to do something good for themselves on a daily basis. I understand that many of us are in relationships which allow little time for individual self-care or incline us to spend all of our non-working moments with a partner. Still, it won't hurt us at least once in a while to get out on our own; there is plenty of time for both solitary self-building and weekly date walks with our partners or social walks with friends or even occasional walks with a community walking club. I would encourage each of us to do all of these things, but suggest we do not completely sacrifice the wonderful sense of personal power and wisdom gained through solitary walking.

Some of the walking exercises I will suggest in a future chapter will require that we be alone in a safe place and walk where we can relax and go into an inner mental space from which we will access states of deep relaxation and insight. We will need to be free of distraction and maintain a strong sense of personal autonomy. If we do choose to do these activities, if we are interested in sharing their effects with others, I would suggest that if we are walking with someone that we and our partner or friend do these exercises separately then get together afterwards to discuss them. For instance, one person could start walking while the other waits five minutes then follows. They meet up at trail's end and share what they have experienced. This can be extremely beneficial. In fact, sharing our walking insights with others, be they about our increased feeling of health and well being or any challenges we face, is a good thing.

Another option available to us is to have a walking partner we don't continually chat with, and with whom we agree to having a silent walking partnership in which we both walk together in silence then use each other as sounding boards to discuss walking benefits once the walk is finished. This is very helpful to both parties. Just be sure that up front you both agree to focus on the mental exercises in this book, turning our focus inward rather than outward, knowing we will have someone with whom to share our thoughts and feelings once our walk is done. Again, this sharing can be incredibly supportive and enlightening.

Some of the benefits of walking alone, at least at times, are as follows. We do not begin to rely on others in order to take our regular walk. I have known some people who would cancel a walk when a walking partner could not go. This is inconsistent with my desire to have each of us take full responsibly for our exercise and health, for to some degree if we only walk when others can walk our walking and health becomes dependent on the choices others make. It is also easy for some to develop a preference for social walking over solitary walking to such a degree that it becomes the only way they will go for a walk.

On the other hand there are some very real benefits in walking with others. It is a great way to develop new or nurture existing relationships, getting together with another and sharing something life-affirming. The same applies to participating in walking clubs where we share the common bond of walking as well as a shared interest in doing something good for ourselves. Many people enjoy and some even need the support of a group to encourage them to walk regularly and to validate their efforts. This can also be a good thing, and in the beginning of this new life change often a necessary thing. Yet, we shouldn't become completely dependent upon it. We, the ones who got ourselves into poor health, are the ones who are responsible for getting us out of it. We don't need others to save us as much as we need to learn how to save ourselves, and the changes we make for ourselves tend to last longer when they are made by us and don't depend too much on the assistance of others.

So how does one strike a balance between these two beneficial but different ways of walking? Do we select walking as a member of a tribe of fellow walkers or select the walk of the solitary warrior, self-reliant, self-motivated, and independent? Once again the answer can be found when we realize that the act of ritualized healthful walking can be viewed as a life metaphor and echoes our human need for both autonomous self-sufficiency and social support. If we are independent solitary types perhaps it would benefit us at times to socialize more with others. And if we are the type who needs constant validation from others to feel valued then perhaps we would benefit greatly by learning to validate ourselves and to be more self-reliant and strong. I would recommend a blended approach, sometimes walking alone and at other times walking with another or in a group. Doing this would not only generate a balance in our lives between self-reliant autonomy and our collective sharing of the life experience with others, but also helps provide the kind of walking variety needed to develop a consistent walking habit. The more we can keep our walking fresh, interesting, and fun, the more we are likely to stay with it. Besides, what really is a good and healthy tribal community but a collection of good and healthy individual warriors?

CHAPTER 11

WARMING UP

It is wise to warm-up and stretch before and after we walk. Warming our muscles, tendons, and joints, bringing blood flow into the areas of our body we intend to work will make our walk more comfortable and help prevent injury. If we begin to walk more briskly as our daily walks progress over time, then we want to walk at a little slower pace at the beginning and end of each walk to warm-up and cool-down more slowly. Some stretching before we start our walk and afterwards is extremely beneficial also. Stretching not only helps to warm muscles but also helps keep muscles from tightening-up after we walk due to their rigorous contraction during exercise.

Here are some stretching exercises we can do. I have adapted them from the National Institutes of Health Weight Control Information Network. Remember, when we stretch we must not hold our breath or bounce and we must do our stretching slowly without any sudden pulls or jerks. Only stretch as far as it is comfortable to do so. Soon, we will begin to notice that this stretching regimen will not only benefit our walking experience but our daily movement and flexibility as well. Do a few of each of the following stretches before and after walking, for it will help us acquire a deeper communication with our bodies and help us sense when each muscle group is sufficiently warmed up.

Side Reach

Reach one arm over your head and down toward the other side. Keep your hips steady and your shoulders level with the arm not being stretched held straight down to your side. Hold for 10 seconds and repeat using your other arm.

Wall Push

Lean your hands on a wall with your feet about three to four feet away from it. Bend one knee and point it toward the wall. Keep your back leg straight with your foot flat and your toes pointed straight ahead. Hold for 10 seconds and repeat with the other leg.

Knee Pull

Lean your back against a wall. Keep your head, hips, and feet in a straight line. Pull one knee to your chest, hold for 10 seconds, then repeat with the other leg.

Leg Curl

Pull your right foot to your buttocks with your right hand. Stand straight and keep your knee pointing straight to the ground. Hold for 10 seconds and repeat with your left foot and hand. Steady yourself with the hand not pulling your foot upward to hold on to something nearby to keep from losing your balance.

Hamstring Stretch

Sit on a sturdy bench or hard surface so that your left leg is stretched out on the bench with your toes pointing up. Keep your right foot flat on the ground. Straighten your back, and when you feel a stretch in the back of your thigh, hold for 10 seconds and repeat with your right leg. If you do not yet feel a stretch, lean forward from your hips until you feel it.

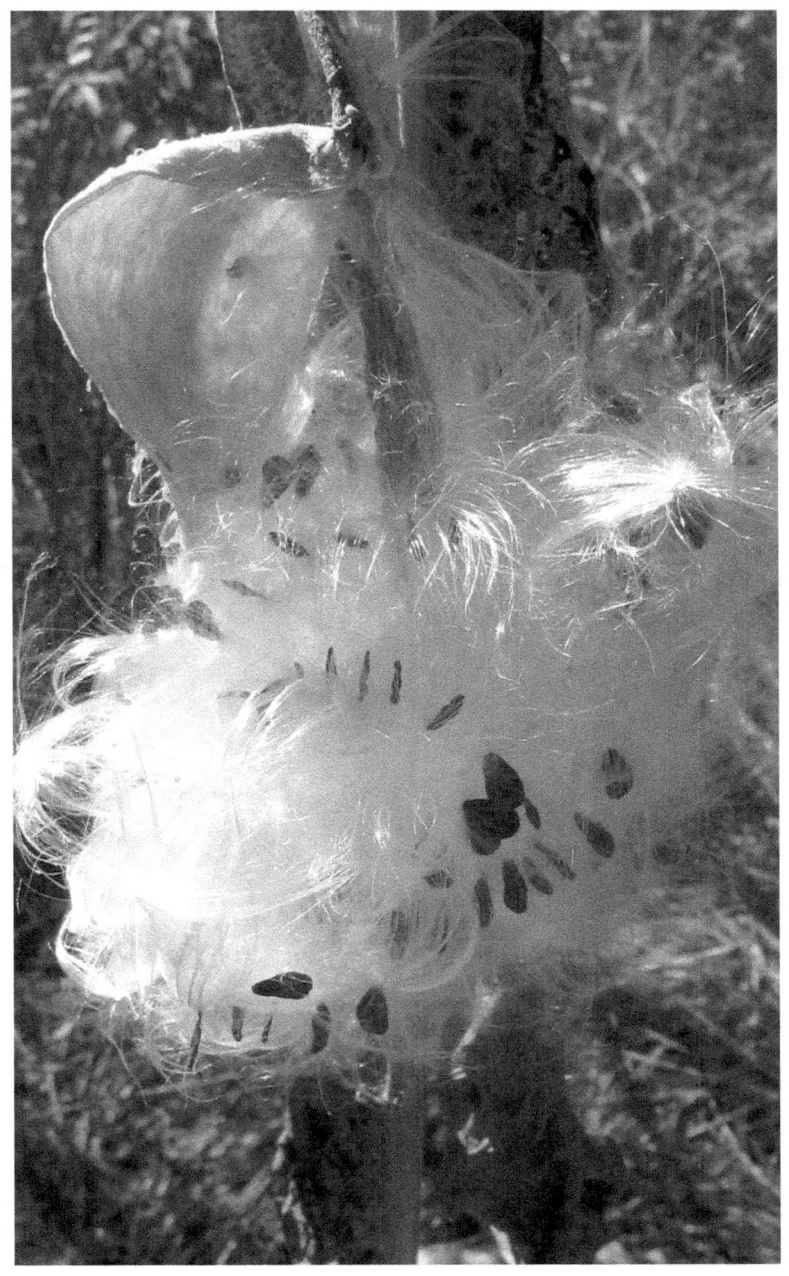

CHAPTER 12

FIRST STEPS

Never underestimate the power of a single step. One step leads to others which together add up to form an extended walk contributing to a life of movement which is wholly transforming. Just as a majestic redwood tree originates from a single seed, a life walk originates and grows from a single step.

It is very important how we start out when trying to develop a consistent walking lifestyle. We must make sure we don't try to do too much too soon or do anything which makes our walks unpleasant, let alone dreaded, but instead makes them something we look forward to, a pleasurable addition to our daily schedule. I believe that it is so important that we walk regularly for the rest of our lives that I encourage you to do whatever it takes in the beginning to insure this happens. If this means starting with baby steps so be it. Each of us alone will know what to do in the beginning because only we know what we are feeling and thinking. I can encourage you and guide you along the way, but in the end each of us on our own will be the one who does the walking. Starting and continuing a walking routine and just how that is accomplished is dependent on each of us as solitary individuals, as is every other choice in life we make. I hope that after you get started that you will take the suggestions I make in this book to get the most from your daily walks, but in the beginning you are largely on your own. Opening the door and stepping out, taking that first step forward and any steps that follow is something I can not do for you.

The first steps we take when we initiate a walking program are a little different for everyone and while I will help when I can, I would not take those first steps for you if I could. I want you to feel the challenge that is involved because I want you to feel the success. And I want you to feel the satisfaction and pride of having done something incredibly beneficial for yourself. I do know one thing, after we have begun to develop a habit of walking regularly it will not be long before we will miss it should we stop. Good health is habit forming, and the way we feel and the results we see will continue to motivate us once we experience them. In much the way that snow builds up slowly in the mountains until at last a tipping-point snow flake falls and an avalanche begins, each step contributes to what can become our own tipping point, a self-actuated cascading movement forward, be it in our daily walk or in our life walk as a whole. In this case that avalanche is our own falling with a gravity-like force down hill into a naturally healthy level of beneficial body movement. We must continue with our walking until we hit our personal tipping point, for after that we are along for one beautiful life-enhancing ride like a sled gliding down a fresh snow-covered slope, and walking becomes a daily pleasure which requires very little effort yet affords immeasurable joy.

My grandson Logan is beginning to walk. He has been moving actively for sometime, rolling around on the floor and crawling here and there. But now he is pulling himself up on things and attempting his first steps. How many steps he will take in his lifetime is unknown and unknowable. While I do not know what the length of his walk will be although I certainly want it to be a long and satisfying one, I do not know how many missteps he will make or how many times he may fall. I hope that he will avoid falling down altogether but that if he does so he will pull himself back to his feet and continue on. I do know that with his first steps he is beginning a long and important journey, the journey which will define his very life, and while the beginning steps are very important, so are those at the end, and each and every step which lies between.

Each daily walk we take is just a smaller version of the life walk. There is even the riddle, "What walks first on four legs, then on two legs, and finally on three?" The answer is of course a human being, because in the beginning of life he crawls, then he walks, and then requires the assistance of a cane in later life. Regardless of how we humans move through life, be it crawling, walking, or hobbling along with the assistance of a cane, we must continue to move or risk not moving at all. When I see my grandson attempting his first steps, I think to myself, "May you move and continue to move for a long time. Walk well, stand proud and keep moving forward, take time to help those you meet along the way and walk for those who are unable to walk, for when you walk you walk for us all."

In one sense when we begin the effort to start walking more, and perhaps even progress to daily walking, we are really just getting out for a little exercise, but as I have suggested before in another sense each walk we take serves as a reminder of the greater walk, the life walk each of us takes. For that reason this book emphasizes both the perspective of the "little walk" and the "big walk" and suggests that they are in fact one and the same. The underlying dynamics of the little walk and the life walk are essentially alike, and for that reason as we improve the quality of our daily walk, we are establishing many skills and habits which will carry over to the bigger walk of life.

As we think about the importance of first steps, it is important not only to warm-up and to stretch but to cultivate an understanding of our goals and intent, and also to develop a proper attitude. Part of that attitude is a respect for the activity we are involved in, having gratitude for being healthy enough to be able to engage in it, and realizing that while it appears to be just a simple routine task it has deeper implications. So here, in this chapter on first steps, I encourage us not only to keep some fundamental and practical things in mind, like warming-up slowly and careful stretching, but to stretch ourselves with an understanding of the really miraculous thing we are doing which may appear to be the simple act of walking but which has a richer meaning beyond that. Once we learn to fully appreciate the gift of walking and give thanks for our ability to participate in it perhaps we then can increase our appreciation of the gift of life itself and give thanks for our ability to participate in it as well. In my view this thankfulness is one of the most natural and fundamental prayers we can express.

CHAPTER 13

WALKING STYLES

Walking styles and speeds vary from person to person. They reflect individual differences in body type, physical conditioning, age and mental attitude. When we first begin a walking regimen, style and speed are not of preeminent importance. In the beginning the goal is simply to walk, to enjoy ourselves, and to keep at it. Initially the number of times we walk per week, the length of time we walk, are also of secondary importance. Our goal at first is to get used to walking on a regular basis and to enjoy getting out into the fresh air and getting away from our daily routine. This is our time for us. Let's enjoy it.

After we have attained this initial goal, we should pat ourselves on the back. If we are getting out to walk 3-5 times per week, and staying out up to a half an hour at a time and have begun already to feel more energetic and look forward to getting out each time, we have accomplished a great deal. In fact, we must stick with it until we do feel that way. Getting into a walking habit, making it consistent, recognizing early changes in the way we feel both physically and mentally is in and of itself a huge accomplishment. Let's attain this first, before we entertain any ideas of altering our walking routine to enhance results.

Another part of our initial goal is getting into a walking habit without trying to do too much too soon. I emphasize again, we don't want to overdo it. If we do so, we may cause injury and soreness to a degree that makes our walking experience distasteful. We don't want distasteful, we want rewarding and fun. If that means doing a little social walking or listening to music on an MP3 player, fine. I would rather see us get out for 10 minutes on every other day taking a relaxing walk with a friend and come home smiling than see us trying to walk a half hour a day at a rapid rate and coming home stiff and sore and having to force ourselves to go out the following day. Get it? The goal is to learn to enjoy the activity of walking and to make it part of our lifestyle. If that takes weeks, months, or years, so be it, but we need to work towards that first.

For most people, it doesn't take long to become habituated to regular walking. Since walking is a natural function of the body, while it may take a little time to get moving again if we have been largely sedentary, the body will be drawn to it. In much the same way as a duck takes to water, a human body takes to movement. Whether we know or not, our bodies have a natural wisdom and are aware of what is in their best interest. Bodies were meant to move, and they know it. So come on in fellow ducks, the water's fine.

Many of us, like myself, have a healthy concern about enhancing our cardiovascular fitness, reducing our blood pressure, and reducing our weight. For those who share that concern we will at some point want to increase the pace at which we walk as well as walk more often and for longer periods of time. But again, even if these are our general goals, we will want to achieve the walking habit first.

I would suggest that once we have established a walking habit we begin to increase the number of times we walk per week up to five days per week first, then increase the length of time we walk up to a minimum of thirty minutes and then work at increasing our speed. After walking consistently for a few months we will most likely already have noticed that our walking pace has increased without our having consciously worked on it to do so. Still, for an even greater cardio work-out we can increase our speed even more, exaggerate our arm swing, or walk occasionally over hilly terrain.

What is the best speed to walk when walking for fitness? Some would say as fast as you can walk, but I remember reading once that a good rule of thumb is walking at about the same pace as the musical pace of the Bee Gee's song *Staying Alive*. It is, as you may remember a rather quick tempoed song and progresses at about 100 beats per minute. That is fortunate because the ideal cardio-walking pace of 100 steps per minute matches it. I recall when I first learned this fact and tried to use the song to increase my pace. I realized that I could not recall the song's lyric's beyond "Staying alive, staying alive," so I looked them up on-line and committed them to memory. It was quite early in the morning and the sun was just coming up over the surrounding mountains as I began my walk the next day. I did not see anyone on the trail where I usually walk and after stretching I walked at my normal pace to warm-up. A few minutes later I rehearsed the lyrics of *Staying Alive* in my head. I almost instantly sped up as I matched my gait to the tempo of the song and moved on down the path quickly. It felt good. I repeated the lyrics again and even spoke them aloud, letting my body fall into the pace of the song's melody. Before I knew it I was really getting into it and I was enjoying singing the lyrics and moving quickly down the trail. Perhaps you remember the beginning scene from Saturday Night Fever where John Travolta is walking down a sidewalk in New York. At the time I could see it clearly in my mind and could almost see myself in The Big Apple prancing down the sidewalk as all heads turned in my direction, and for a moment I felt as confident and painfully attractive as Travolta. As I continued down my walking path I decided to really let loose, feeling my body relax into the pulsing rhythm of the music and singing even louder, accentuating my gait to match Travolta's cocky walking style. I began to sing freely out loud.

"Well, you can tell by the way I use my walk,
I'm a woman's man—no time to talk.
Music loud and women warm, I've been kicked around
Since I was born.
And now it's all right. It's OK.
And you may look the other way.
We can try to understand
The New York Times' effect on man.

Whether you're a brother or whether you're a mother,
You're stayin' alive, stayin' alive.
Feel the city breakin' and everybody shakin', people,
Stayin' alive, stayin' alive.
Ah, ha, ha, ha, stayin' alive, stayin' alive.
Ah, ha, ha, ha, stayin' alive.

As I did my best to imitate the brothers Gibb nasal singing style, my head tilted back, my knees lifting high, I began to sense a presence to my left. A woman jogger came running past me from behind just as I got to the part of the song, "You can tell by the way I use my walk, I'm a ladies man … no time to talk…" The woman quickly jetted past me, turned her head for a second in my direction, smiled uncomfortably at me then gave me a thumbs up before speeding ahead. I felt the blood rush to my face.

To be honest I am a little more careful now about singing aloud during my walks, for the sake of both myself and others. Still, I do encourage us all to vary both the speed of our walking and the variety of inclines on which we walk. Each speed and incline alternative we try works our muscles in a unique way, and those muscles include our heart muscle. It is good at times to push ourselves at a little faster pace and if we begin to feel fatigued then we slow our pace down to catch our breath before speeding up again.

PART 2

WALKING
THE MIND

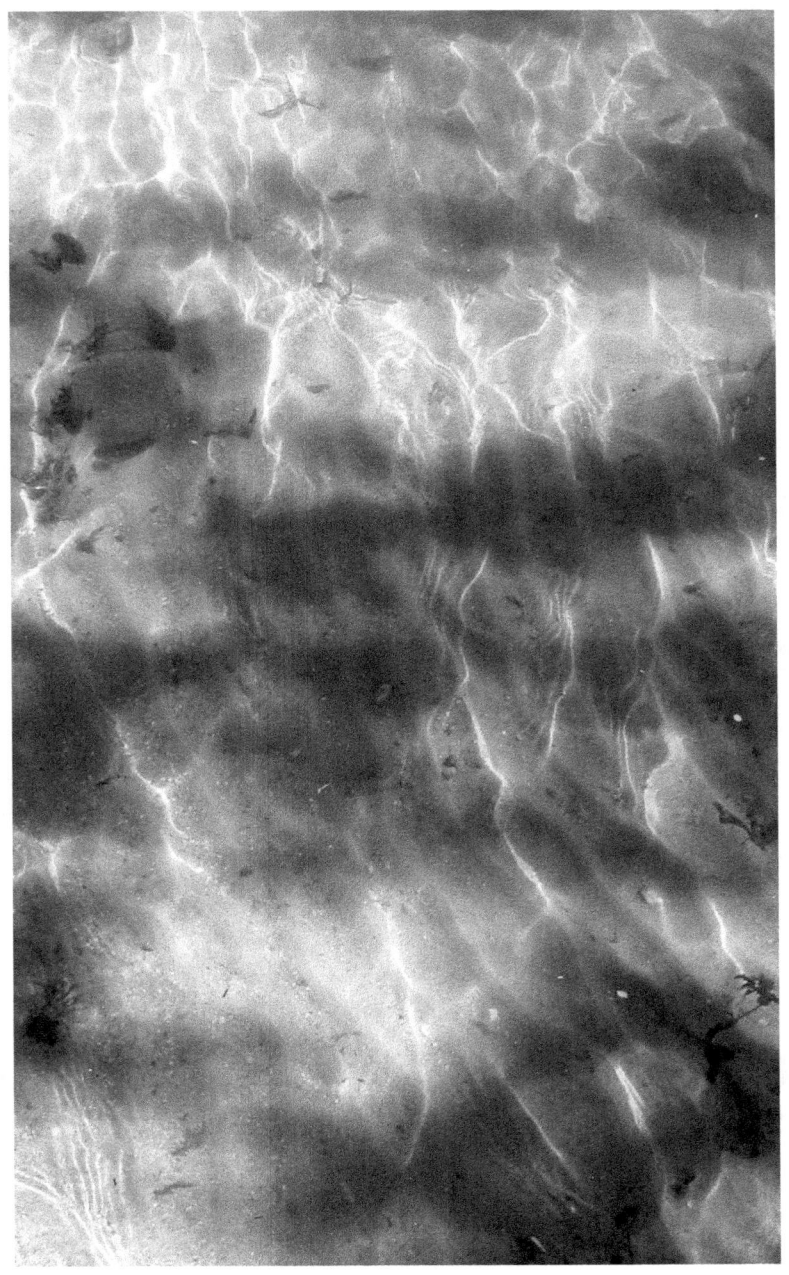

CHAPTER 14

LISTENING TO OUR BODY AND OUR MIND

Once we have become comfortable with our new walking regimen, found a way to make it a regular part of our daily activity, and have converted any sitting inertia we may have had into movement inertia, the rate at which we progress is up to each of us. Let's be clear first of all as to what progress in our walking program means. Let's define it as the movement toward achieving the goal of walking consistently and slowly increasing the pace and duration of our walks. Let's think of progress in this program also as simply feeling better, having more energy, and being generally happier. When we see these goals starting to be realized will depend upon a schedule only each of us can determine. Still, there is no rush to get anywhere, for wherever we are in our activity level after we have started walking, it is better than where we were before we began. We need to realize that by just starting a regular walking program we are making progress and advancing. Every single step we take is an advancement bringing us closer to better health, and that step is its own destination and accomplishment. In a sense every step we take now gives us an additional step later, for some have suggested that for each minute we walk now an additional minute is added to our lives.

We will find that even while we are beginning to move toward some imagined ideal consistent work-out routine we are already experiencing dramatic changes. In physical terms we are beginning to lose excess weight, increasing our cardiovascular fitness, feeling much more energetic, and developing a sense of well-being. It is surprising how quickly we progress in this way and begin to feel better, largely because we never realized that we hadn't been feeling all that great for some time.

One of the greatest benefits we will quickly gain from regular walking will be a closer relationship to both our bodies and minds. Our bodies and minds will actually seem nearer to us than before because we will have an increased capacity to hear them much more clearly, and they will begin to have more to say. But don't be surprised if in the beginning our minds and bodies have difficulty working together and seem somewhat alienated from each other. Due to cultural forces and personal choices, what should be our mind/body synthesis is largely fractured and ineffective. It will take time and effort for it to heal. Because we have recently lived more and more inside our heads and preferred screen time to time inside our own bodies, the once healthy communication between our bodies and minds has deteriorated to a great degree. The more we live in our heads the less we live in our bodies, and the more difficult it is to reach a state of holistic mind/body integration. The rift we will find between the our minds and bodies is, I believe, a unique modern form of what the psychological community calls "bodily disassociation", a detachment of the mind from the body.

Traditionally defined, bodily disassociation is caused by a severe trauma to the body, but today there is a disassociation from the body caused by voluntarily choosing to spend more time in our heads to the exclusion of our bodies. I refer to this as "voluntary bodily dissociation" and it results in an injury to both body and mind, for to have optimal health both mind and body must work closely together. Even though traumatic bodily dissociation and voluntary bodily dissociation originate in very different ways, the dynamics are similar and what we learn from one we can easily apply to the other.

I find the terms "body awareness" and "bodily dissociation" best defined in a paper found in PMC, a journal published by the U.S. National Institutes of Health's National Library of Medicine. It is found in a paper titled 'Measuring Dimensions of Body Connection: Body Awareness and Bodily Dissociation' by Cynthia Price, Ph.D. and Elaine Thompson, Ph.D. Here is a quote from the paper's abstract.

"Body awareness and bodily dissociation, often not clearly defined, are discrete but experientially linked concepts. Body awareness is multifaceted. It involves sensory awareness—the ability to identify and experience inner sensations of the body (e.g., a tight muscle) and the overall emotional/physiologic state of the body (e.g., relaxed, tense). Body awareness also involves attending to bodily information in daily life, noticing bodily changes/responses to emotion and/or environment. The concept of bodily dissociation is characterized by avoidance of internal experience. Bodily dissociation has experiential aspects including normal everyday experiences, such as distraction from bodily experience;

this dissociation also includes the experience of separation from bodily experience or bodily self, and emotional disconnection—difficulty with identifying, expressing, and attending to emotion."

Our goal will be to gain through walking greater body awareness and to eliminate bodily disassociation caused by the mind's voluntary detachment from the body. In my own walking experience, I have learned that if not the ringleader, that the ego is at least a willing accomplice in that abandonment and a noisy apologist for our mind's flight from somatic wisdom. For our purposes here, we think of the ego as that self-appointed voice inside our heads, the one we constantly hear talking and which we confuse with being the totality of our mind's awareness and of somehow being the person we truly are. Many people know no other aspect of mind than this. And this usurpation of the whole mind by the ego, and it's new obsession with the artificial technology-based stimulations of culture which arise outside of the body has led in part not only to an evolving narcissistic culture but to the ever-widening mind/body split.

The result of this split is an injury which is numbing to our psychophysical awareness and the symptoms of this injury while fortunately not usually as severe as traumatic bodily disassociation are eerily similar. In both cases one may experience depression, anxiety and panic attacks, mood swings, headaches, sleep disorders, phobias, alcohol and drug abuse, eating disorders, obsessive-compulsive behavior and various physical health problems. And in severe cases a person can experience something called "fragmented identity" where an alternate personality begins to control our behavior, thoughts and feelings. In my view that personality is our renegade ego which more and more often runs roughshod over the body or ignores it all together.

Again, the trauma we experience through our exposure to daily stress, by ignoring the needs of our bodies, and by living mostly in our heads to the exclusion of the body, may never reach the levels of severity we find in body disassociation due to body trauma, but the symptoms listed above should serve as warning signs if we experience any of them. So, does consistent walking actually help if we have any of these symptoms or help to keep them from developing in the future? We have already discovered the answer to that question by learning that walking and other forms of exercise are currently used to successfully treat and prevent some of these problems, and I maintain that with consistent walking integrated with mental exercises designed to put our minds back in touch with our bodies we can not only combat these symptoms but help to heal the mind/body split itself. After all, we can see just by viewing people on the street today that mind/body splits are ubiquitous. Three quarters of the bodies we see walking about are overweight and unfit, and they waddle through life as the distracted mind looks the other way and holds the latest gadget to its ear. If our minds were truly in touch with our bodies could something like this happen? It should prove to us that the problem our society faces in this regard is not just a physical one but a mental one as well, for how could a mind attuned to the body watch its own physical embodiment destroy itself and shorten the duration of its life? When I see large groups of large people in public now and see how more and more of us wear coats of fat which insulate and isolate us from the world, I think of the title of Stanley Keleman's fine book, *Your Body speaks Its Mind*.

It is easy for us all to get distracted from the wisdom of our own bodies and cease to question the credibility of the voice which continually talks inside our heads. Over the years we have taken both for granted, assuming we must already be closely in touch with them when in truth we were not. Walking will help change this. Because walking attunes us more closely to our physical selves and forces us to attend more closely to our thoughts since we have plenty of time to observe them throughout our walks, we will begin to see, often for the first time, how we actually interact with and respond not only to our own body's communication but to the world body which surrounds us. The reason for this is that our mind's relationship with our own material body is similar to our mind's relationship with the material world at large, for what really is the world but the material body in which we live and our own thoughts an attempt to understand what that world means? Could our ignoring of the growing environmental disaster which surrounds us be related to the mind's growing neglect of the body, be it our own body or the world body in which we live?

The pace of 21st Century living with its constant distractions and exposure to unnatural stress, its focus on imaginary virtual realities as opposed to traditional physical realities has numbed many of us to the workings of our own biology. People get ill and don't even sense it until it progresses to a serious level, others continue to wear themselves out while their own bodies are begging them to slow down and rest. One of the greatest benefits of regular exercise is a reattuning of the mind to the body's wisdom, and it can have deep and significant implications with great benefits to our physical and mental health. One of those benefits is that our minds not only learn to share a deeper connection with our body but develop a closer connection with the natural world. This happens in part because our bodily senses heighten as we walk and our mind's awareness of those senses heighten as well. Soon, after you begin your walking program, you too will feel it and soon be happily telling others about the remarkable new relationship you are in, an intimate relationship with your very own body and mind.

Why does our body suddenly seem to speak-up when we begin to walk? Here is what I have learned in my own walking program. It is because our bodies naturally speak-up when there is a major change in what we ask of it, particularly during a change as radical as moving from a nearly sedentary lifestyle to a lifestyle of increased movement. Think of an iron gate's loud squeaking when it hasn't been used or oiled for sometime and then is suddenly asked to work. With increased movement comes a new level of communication with our bodies. Our listening minds will be compelled to pay attention to what our bodies are saying and learn to interpret what they say, and learn also to discriminate between serious complaints of the whole mind and the more trivial complaints of ego.

For instance, while it is normal to be sore when we use muscles we have ignored for a while and to feel a little "healthy tired" when we start to exercise more than normal, our minds will have to learn to tell the difference between appropriate levels of soreness and fatigue from those which signal that we need to ease off some in our workouts. We can usually make this determination by the levels of discomfort we feel; a little soreness and fatigue is normal, a lot is not. We need to work through the low levels, but ease off if we experience high levels. Remember, a body that has been at rest wants to stay at rest and it will protest a little when we ask it to become more active. But pushing our body too soon, too hard, will lead to possible injury and a fatigue which is unhealthful, so we must learn to tell the difference and take precautions accordingly. Again, it will take time for the mind to reestablish a renewed and healthy communication with our body. Undoubtedly at one time our bodies and minds communicated in a close and natural way, but they are now a bit like an old married couple who have quit talking to each other because they think they know what the other will say, leaving the body to lounge by itself on the sofa as the mind sits alone in a recliner and watches T.V.

It is not just complaints of the body our minds must listen for but for positive feedback as well. After only a few walks we will begin to notice positive changes in the way we feel. While it may seem counter intuitive, expending a little more energy than we are used to often makes us feel like we have more energy to expend. It is important to note the way adding more movement to our lives effects our sleep patterns and our overall mood also. In other words, while both our bodies and our minds will make it easier for us to hear them because of walking, we need to learn to listen to what our bodies have to say fully and deeply, both its complaints and compliments twenty-four hours a day and not just when we are walking. By closely monitoring what we are feeling and thinking we will learn not only the appropriate times to make adjustments to our walking routine and when to continue as normal, but when to celebrate the many positive changes we become aware of and allow them to encourage us as we walk.

Because our bodies and minds are interwoven, an unhealthy body can make the mind sick, and unhealthy mind can make the body sick. Something like depression can be hurtful not just to our mental state but to our bodies as well, just as a sick, diseased, and lethargic body can be extremely detrimental to our mental health. For that reason we pay close attention not only to what our bodies are saying but track our mind's response to them. While it is relatively easy to know when we are not feeling well physically, it is more difficult to know when we are not thinking well, or when the thoughts inside our own heads are actually helping to make us ill. And it is difficult also to tell the difference between the wisdom of our whole minds and the endless concerns and spin-doctoring of the hyperactive voice of ego.

Why would our own thinking make us ill? It is because since our minds abandoned our bodies they have developed some negative habits. Not only have they lost their physical mooring, they have sailed away from somatic intelligence, the inherent wisdom of the body. Rather than thinking more deeply and holistically our frantic stressed-out egos have taken over the driver's seat inside our heads and communicate the toxic messages of doubt and fear, fast-paced living, and divisiveness they have learned in the world outside the body. While we want our whole minds to rejoin the body, our egos are not the whole mind, and it is important to monitor what our ego minds are thinking and to carefully separate the toxic thoughts from those which promote wellness. In other words, initially as we reintegrate the mind back into the body, our egos will be on probation, and we will supervise them carefully and teach them healthier ways to think .

While we will call the voice inside our heads our ego, we will call the one who listens to the thoughts inside our head our "inner witness," and it is that part of our minds we will want to emphasize while walking. We will learn to use our inner witness to oversee and control what our ego is telling us and learn how to stifle any thoughts which keep us stuck in a morass of negative thinking and encourage it to focus instead on thoughts which aid our progression to better health, thoughts which are health-affirming and not those which are health-negating.

In the following chapters of this book we will learn how to retrain our minds to do this. We will learn a variety of mental exercises which will help promote relaxation, peace of mind, positive attitude and inner harmony. We will soon discuss the importance of positive thinking, learn how to use affirmations and meditations, and discover that changes to our mental state will be as dramatic as those to our physical state. But for now, when I talk about watching for changes in our mental state I am talking about something more basic. In the early stages of our walking I want us to start to witness for ourselves the connection between psyche and soma, between the health of our body and the health of our mind. I want us to start to see how daily walking impacts our brains and bodies in a very real and beneficial way. Some of these changes are subtle, so pay close attention. In fact, start on the day you begin walking by making at least one weekly journal entry regarding what you are learning about your mind/body connection.

There are more details at the back of this book in Appendix 1 on how to record the new dialogue we will share with our newly evolving healthy minds and bodies and the importance of doing so. And it bears repeating, as we develop our listening skills it will seem as if our bodies and minds start to speak to us louder and more succinctly, but in fact we hear that best for which we listen. Our minds and bodies are not just speaking louder, we are being more attentive. Over time we will advance to a point where our minds and bodies speak with nearly the same voice, and when one is happy and fulfilled the other is happy and fulfilled as well. We will learn to discern too between the ego's chatty rhetoric and the whole mind's deeper thoughts and wisdom.

Later in this book we will discuss ways to tell the difference between the wisdom of our deeper self and that brain voice we know so well, but for now, know that there is a difference and recognize that through this new walking regimen our mental health is tied to our physical health and is of equal importance. Let's now look at what I call "inner walking" and some of the mental benefits of exercise and specifically of walking.

CHAPTER 15

INNER WALKING

I once knew a man who worked very hard so that one day he would have the time and money to take his dream vacation. Even while working in his office he often found himself turning to look out the window behind his desk imagining a South Sea's island in the distance with a hammock where he swayed in blissful peacefulness beneath the soaring palms. The more he daydreamed about this on-going fantasy the more frantically he worked. He rushed around his office, a phone planted in his ear, then hurried to meetings as he barked orders to his secretary and strove to meet daily deadlines in order to please his superiors. He stayed at work late every evening getting that one last thing done then fought the freeway traffic on his drive home as visions of palm trees still swayed his head.

Eventually my friend found time for a trip to Tahiti. Of course when he arrived there he made sure that he had internet service so he could check in with the office and purchased the local Tahitian cell phone service just in case there was an emergency back home that required his attention. For he was after all a very responsible man and shared in the delusion many of us share, the delusion that we are indispensable. As he sat in a lounge chair next to the resort's pool with a small paper umbrella in the drink on the table next to him, he looked out at the beautiful turquoise water and the palm trees slowly waving overhead. Finally, his dream had come true. But after about fifteen minutes of tropical bliss he began to get restless. He found himself thinking about some of the work projects he had left unfinished on his desk, and wondered if his business partner was reviewing them. As he looked out over the beautiful water spread out before him, he was suddenly transported back to his office where he could see in detail his desk and furniture and his business partner bent over and perusing a stack of his papers. And he could even see the large picture window in his office where he once looked out toward the distant horizon and imagined himself to be on the very island where he now sat.

In the end, while my friend had at last transported his physical body to his dream destination, his mind was still back at the office. It was as if he had forgotten to pack his brain and had left it switched on and sitting on his desk at home. Unfortunately it did not get any better. Instead of his exotic vacation being a relaxing break for body and mind from the stresses and worries of his working life it only made things worse. Back home when he worried he could do something about it, call someone or tell someone what to do, but on an island on the other side of the world he could do nothing, and now he had not only the same worries he had before, he had the frustration of feeling powerless to do anything about them. Regardless of how hard he tried, my friend could not get work out of his head, and what he once thought of as paradise became a kind of living hell.

The concept of inner walking is based on the clear understanding that the body and mind are interconnected. There is an old adage in walking circles, "If you want to know if someone has a flabby mind, feel their legs." Walkers learn quickly that a healthier body leads to a healthier mind. Change one, we change the other. While this change occurs to some extent without even trying, we can with a little effort greatly increase the speed of our progression to better mental health if we work diligently to alleviate unhealthy habits of mind as we walk.

As we walk toward increased health it is important that we do not undermine our efforts by holding onto the unhealthy habits of mind. It is important to engage in a kind of "brain washing" which in this case literally means cleaning up our mental state while simultaneously working to develop healthier physical behaviors. It's worth repeating Dr. William B. Stewart's insight, "Everything we think, feel, say, and do is either health creating or health negating. Everything." For those of us who walk and who practice inner mental walking techniques, there are several important lessons in the story I have related about my friend on vacation in the South Pacific. One is that we create habitual behaviors not only in our bodies but also in our minds, another is that many of these habits are hurtful and difficult to break. Still another is that if we recognize that the body and the mind are deeply intertwined we know that as we break the bad habits of the inactive body we must also break the bad habits of a mind which has become debilitated with worries, stress, and continual mental chatter. These are the toxins of the mind, comparable to the toxins of our bodies, and we need to rid ourselves of both. In this book our walking regimen will work not only toward contributing to a healthy shift from inactivity to activity for our bodies, it will also work to shift our minds away from negative and obsessive thoughts which lead to increased anxiety and stress and create instead a mind at peace which is filled with positive thoughts and greater joy.

Long ago the Greek philosopher Hippocrates said, "Walking is the medicine of man." And today we know that a walking routine not only slows the rate at which we age and helps in the prevention of disease, it can also help put our minds in a better state of health. Mental stress whether generated by outside events or self-created can have dramatic and detrimental effects on the body, both in slowing the body's natural healing abilities but also in actually making the body more receptive to illness. Body health and mental health go hand in hand. If my friend had been able to take his mind as well as his body on a vacation to Tahiti it would have become the dream vacation he imagined it would be.

In a 2007 article in the Journal of American Medicine, Dr. Sheldon Cohen and collaborators found through reviewing current research on the topic that stress contributed significantly to the development of disease. It does so in two different ways, one is that people under stress tend not to sleep well or eat right, exercise less and smoke more, and do not get sufficient medical treatment when needed. The second way is the direct effect stress has on the human body. Stress affects the endocrine system which releases hormones that influence other biological systems, including the immune system. "Effects of stress on regulation of immune and inflammatory processes have the potential to influence depression, infectious, autoimmune, and coronary artery disease, and at least some (e.g., viral) cancers," the authors write.

What is of particular interest in this article is the way it reveals the relation of stress to depression and then how depression relates to illness and disease. While Cohen says that "social stressors" such as the death of a loved one and divorce are the biggest causes of depression, chronic stress such as stress experienced routinely in the workplace contributes to cardiovascular illnesses such as coronary heart disease, a fact clearly demonstrated in many of the medical studies they reviewed.

Sources of stress, types of stress, and degrees of stress vary greatly, and since every individual responds to stress differently, what affects one person may not affect another. While the effects of major stressors on the body and health of individual are more obvious, we are just beginning to learn the effect that so called "minor stressors" can have particularly when we are exposed to them for extensive periods of time. At one time in our history low level radiation was thought to be harmless. There were x-ray machines at shoe stores so you could look through your shoes to see if your toes were too crowded, and at the time it was thought that any number of medical x-rays could be taken without any hurtful impact. We know differently now. I believe we will come to believe the same of low-level stress and that eventually we will do more and more to mitigate the effects of all types and levels of stress from our lives, be it low level or high. While a certain amount of stress has been part of the human experience since time immemorial and can have some benefits under specific situations of fight or flight, the unrelenting stress we currently experience as a part of daily modern life is unprecedented, unnatural, and over time extremely hurtful.

One of the most subtle and less obvious forms of stress which affects our mental state is mind stress. To a great degree mind stress is self-generated. This often makes it difficult for us to see because we are so close to it, but on the positive side, because we ourselves create it, we also have the ability to rid ourselves of it. The basic forms of mind stress fall under the three basic categories of: negative thinking, worry, and constant interior mental chatter. All three of these mental negatives can be habitual, and the more habitual they become the more detrimental they are to both mind and body. As I stated earlier, many of these bad habits have been assimilated by the ego aspect of mind which it has learned while participating in, navigating through, and surviving the daily pressures of modern living. Watch for yourself and witness the harmful habits of your own mind. How much time do you spend thinking negatively about the events of your life, about yourself, or constantly worrying about what might happen? Does it help?

Much of our negative thinking is generated due to the fact that we spend most of our time interacting with a world which is fast-paced, media-driven, and filled with endless stories of how things are falling apart and with constant advertising hype telling us how we are falling short in relation to those around us. The goal of course is to sell us something that makes us more acceptable and loveable to everyone else. It is very difficult to maintain mental focus and balance in an environment which is constantly harping on the negative, the short-comings of human life and the short-comings of us as individuals and our lives as well. No wonder many people once they get off work don't feel like coming home for a life-affirming walk but turn instead to a good stiff drink.

With perpetual negative thinking comes low self-esteem and with low self-esteem comes worry. We worry about the craziest things, "Will we make enough money? Will our kids be as smart and get as good an education as all of their friends? Are our teeth white enough? Our clothes of the latest style?" To a great extent we have become so numbed to these constant and sometimes subtle forms of mind manipulation and external message bombardment that we are no longer conscious of them and have gotten used to them, assuming they are a normal part of living in the 21st century. Most of us are not aware of the toll they take on us mentally and thereby on our health in general. Most of us are not aware either of the fundamental effect our general environment has on us or how it impacts our well-being, and in this case by general environment I mean in part the frenetic speed at which the world moves around us, particularly if we live in a city setting. We may not always hear the cars passing outside, the planes passing overhead, the T.V. on and blaring in the next room, or the clocks endlessly tick-tocking all around the house. We may have learned to tune them out, yet still they find their way into every recess of our being and subliminally affect our stress levels, and thereby affect our health. In other words, the human organism responds to these things whether we are conscious of them or not.

If I were to tell you that current scientific research shows that people who live in larger cites actually walk at a faster pace than people who live in smaller ones would you believe it? It's true, for whether we realize it or not we sense the general life pace around us and adjust our walking pace to match it. This "pace of our surroundings" also affects the mental pace which keeps us hopping between our daily tasks and the pace at which we move between each thought inside our heads.

A person living out in the country lives in an environment which is not only more slowly paced but one which also provides more "mind time" for reflection and contemplation, and for thinking through each thought. And because things happen more slowly in a rural setting people move more slowly and are not only able to stay with a single thought for a longer period of time but find it much easier to slip between their thoughts to appreciate the depth of the present moment and the world in which it exists. City dwellers, not so much. Their thoughts are numerous and fast-paced, allowing little time for experiencing anything else, let alone for time to feel the pleasure of simple being. The city mind is busier with thoughts which are generally of less depth, more numerous and unceasing. Hindus refer to this constant parade of rapid and shallow thoughts inside our heads as "the sound of the drunken monkey," and in their own culture have established methods to quiet the noisy primate down. Listen to the hodgepodge of thoughts inside your own head for a few minutes to understand why the term "drunken monkey" is appropriate. If you were able to somehow record the inner monologue of your ego which runs inside your head, and play it back, you would be astounded at the voice's general message and dynamic. There are so many expressions of worry and concern, so much scattered focus and superficiality driven by hyper-emotional and illogical thinking. As we walk, our intent is not so much to eradicate the voice of ego but to listen to it objectively. If we are going to be influenced by what it has to say then we need to question its beliefs and conclusions, then choose which thoughts we allow to stay, those which support our greater health.

While walking we need to at least try to get our inner monkey under control. In the beginning, at the very least we should try to learn to focus for a time on one positive mental topic at a time or focus on an external sensual attractor we are drawn to in our current walking environment, the sounds of birds fluttering in the trees, our own unique pattern of breathing, the sun moving behind a cloud. We must focus on <u>one</u> thing and stay with it, and think of it as a choice of either controlling our inner monkey or letting our inner monkey control us. If we don't like the drunken monkey analogy, perhaps we might think of gaining control of our inner monologue as taming a wild stallion, our own mind running wild like a mustang as it flees a civilization filled with city thought and reflexive worry while our internal inner witness stays calm and attempts to settle the wild horse down playing the role of "mind whisperer", making sure that in the end we will be able to ride our minds rather than allow our minds to ride us.

The materialistic, commodity-filled world in which most of us live, driven by commerce and the need for social acceptance and running at a hectic speed where it is difficult to catch our breaths or to get a thought in edge-wise, is not a new one. While it is getting worse by the day, there were those who saw it coming and warned society about its detrimental impact to living a meaningful life. As early as the mid 1800's Transcendentalist writers Ralph Waldo Emerson and Henry David Thoreau both expressed a deep concern for mankind and his ever-growing disassociation from the natural world, as well as our society's evolving attachment to material things. It was Emerson who said of our society's mounting materialism, "Things are in the saddle, and they ride mankind."

In his writings Thoreau was often emphasizing the distinction between the city and woods while he lived alone at Walden Pond and took long daily walks through the surrounding forests. For him city life and its inherent lifestyle represented the separation of man from the wilderness, from its qualities of freedom, spontaneity, and natural wisdom, and thereby stifled the development of those qualities within mankind itself. In his short essay *Walking,* Thoreau makes his feelings clear,

"I think that I cannot preserve my health and spirits, unless I spend four hours a day at least---and it is commonly more than that---sauntering through the woods and over the hills and fields, absolutely free from all worldly engagements. You may safely say, 'A penny for your thoughts, or a thousand pounds.' When sometimes I am reminded that the mechanics and shopkeepers stay in their shops not only all the forenoon, but all the afternoon too, sitting with crossed legs, so many of them---as if the legs were made to sit upon, and not to stand or walk upon---I think that they deserve some credit for not having all committed suicide long ago."

Thoreau's belief of man's disassociation from nature corresponds closely to the mind's disassociation from the body and the destructive influence that can have on our mental and physical health. For that reason I would encourage you when possible to walk in a natural setting, be it a city park or the countryside. The concrete cityscape is too closely attached to the very things we are seeking relief from, meaningless non-directed mental chatter, largely of a negative kind, and somewhat artificial lives whose meaning is measured by the incessant ticking of the clock. We are searching for peace of mind and the simple elegant joys found more easily in the non-mechanized and natural, in the deepest heart of nature be it a park or old growth forest, or even the renewing forest which lies within each of us, our own inner nature. Regardless, one thing is sure, wherever we take our walks we will leave our city thoughts behind and yield to the joy of simple grounded being and hear Thoreau's words, "What business have I in the woods, if I am thinking of something out of the woods?"

CHAPTER 16

COMBATING DEPRESSION, STRESS, ANXIETY, AND BUILDING SELF-ESTEEM

As I have suggested in previous chapters because our minds are deeply connected to our bodies it is possible to improve our physical health through improving our mental health and improve our mental health by improving our physical health. In the next chapter we will discuss ways to work specifically on our mental health while we walk, an effort which benefits not only our minds but our bodies as well. But first let's look at some of the studies and research which help reveal the mind/body interdependence in cases where exercise is used in the treatment of mental disorders like stress, anxiety and depression. This information will help us understand why many people may begin their regular walking routine because of its numerous benefits to their physical health and appearance but it becomes in most cases its mental benefits which keeps people lacing-up their walking shoes. Yes, you will feel better physically and reduce your susceptibility to disease, slow the effects of aging, and lose weight, but it will be the way you feel emotionally and mentally that will keep you walking day in and day out, month in and month out, year in and year out. Again, physical health and mental health are closely intertwined: we feel better mentally when we feel better physically in part because we have much more energy and are less lethargic. Still, consistent walking has effects directly on the brain itself independently of other physical benefits and has been shown in many studies to be effective in reducing the three most prevalent mental ailments: stress, anxiety and depression.

An article in the August 6, 2010 issue of *Science Daily* magazine states, "Exercise is a magic drug for many people with depression and anxiety disorders, and it should be more widely prescribed by mental health care providers, according to researchers who analyzed the results of numerous published studies." The article goes on to discuss what they refer to as a "meta-analysis" of research literature in this area and concludes:

"The research literature suggests that for many variables there is now ample evidence that a definite relationship exists between exercise and improved mental health. This is particularly evident in the case of a reduction of anxiety and depression. For these topics, there is now considerable evidence derived from over hundreds of studies with thousands of subjects to support the claim that "exercise is related to a relief in symptoms of depression and anxiety."

In the article's summary the authors also note, "At the present time, it appears that aerobic exercise enhances physical self-concept and self-esteem, but more research needs to be done to confirm these initial findings."

Likewise, a report in *Research Digest* by Dr. Daniel M. Landers from Arizona State University concludes, "We now have evidence to support the claim that exercise is related to positive mental health as indicated by relief in symptoms of depression and anxiety."

"Exercise has been shown to have tremendous benefits for mental health," says Jasper Smits, director of the Anxiety Research and Treatment Program at Southern Methodist University. "The more therapists who are trained in exercise therapy, the better off patients will be…Individuals who exercise report fewer symptoms of anxiety and depression, and lower levels of stress and anger," Smits says. "Exercise appears to affect, like an antidepressant, particular neurotransmitter systems in the brain, and it helps patients with depression re-establish positive behaviors. For patients with anxiety disorders, exercise reduces their fears and related bodily sensations such as a racing heart and rapid breathing." After patients have passed a health assessment, Smits says they should work up to the public health dose of needed exercise which is 150 minutes a week of moderate-intensity activity or 75 minutes a week of vigorous-intensity activity. At a time when 40 % of Americans are sedentary, he says, mental health care providers can serve as their patients' exercise guides and motivators.

Learning from the Sound of Our Own Footsteps: Building Self-esteem

When we take our shoes for a walk just what is the sound of walking? It is a sound like a metronome's which provides the fundamental rhythm playing behind all of life's music. It echoes the sound of the heart beating, the body's constant reminder that we are alive, but which also reminds us that time is passing. It is the sound of our movement through time and space, the sound of our own unique identity revealing itself. It is the repeating proclamation that we are worthy of being cared for and making time for, and the sound that signifies that we are vitally alive and at the center of something very magical: our own lives.

The information from the research texts above suggests that the evidence is clear, regular exercise helps reduce anxiety and depression. And since we know that depression can contribute to the development of illness as well as be a symptom of illness it is easy to see the correlation between our mental state and our physical health. Still there is another mental benefit of exercise for us beyond the reduction of anxiety and stress which is suggested in the articles cited above. That is the relationship between our mental and physical health and our level of self-esteem.

We are learning more and more about the relationship between low self-esteem, depression and the compulsive/addictive disorders people develop to self-medicate them. The dynamics of the downward spiral associated with self-abusive behaviors meant to temporarily escape depression but which in the end only increase that depression is well documented. If we can better understand how low self-esteem creates a sense of inner emptiness which many people feel and then attempt to fill with a variety of addictive and compulsive behaviors then perhaps we can stop the development of that terribly destructive dynamic within ourselves. The article I emphasize below, written by the journal's staff, is taken from Oxford Journal's

Health Education Research, vol. 19, no. 4. Oxford University Press. Here is a segment of the paper's abstract.

"This paper stresses the importance of self-esteem as a protective factor and a non-specific risk factor in physical and mental health. Evidence is presented illustrating that self-esteem can lead to better health and social behavior, and that poor self-esteem is associated with a broad range of mental disorders and social problems, both internalizing problems (e.g. depression, suicidal tendencies, eating disorders and anxiety) and externalizing problems (e.g. violence and substance abuse). We discuss the dynamics of self-esteem in these relations."

We all talk about self-esteem and recognize its importance particularly in the development of children. We know that it is crucial for kids to develop a positive self-image both physically and mentally, yet often times we fail to think of it in relation to our adult lives. We assume that the development of self-esteem is something we have worked through in the past, something which is somehow already established in our psyches and something we no longer need to be conscious of, let alone continue to be mindful of and persist in developing. I think of self-esteem as if it were just another muscle in the mind/body synthesis, one which needs continual exercise to stay strong and free of atrophy. The way we see ourselves like everything else changes over time and can be dramatically modified by both internal and external forces and for this reason we must continually monitor our self-esteem and plan specific activities which bolster it and make sure we continually engage in mental habits which affirm it. When it comes to our self-esteem we need to be constantly mindful of it and consistently nurture it, for as the following quote from our article suggests, the way in which we either esteem ourselves or do not esteem ourselves ultimately determines who we are.

"The beliefs and evaluations people hold about themselves determine who they are, what they can do and what they can become (Burns, 1982). These powerful, inner influences provide an internal guiding mechanism, steering and nurturing individuals through life, and governing their behavior. People's concepts and feelings about themselves are generally labeled as their self-concept and self-esteem. These, together with their ability to deal with life's challenges and to control what happens to them, are widely documented in literature (Seligman, 1975; Bandura, 1977; Bowlby, 1980; Rutter, 1992; Harter, 1999)."

The internal guidance mechanism of self-esteem, not only steers us through life, away from self-injuring and even self-destructive behaviors, but can also guide us toward a happier and more fulfilling life.

"Empirical studies over the last 15 years indicate that self-esteem is an important psychological factor contributing to health and quality of life (Evans, 1997). Recently, several studies have shown that subjective well-being significantly correlates with high self-esteem, and that self-esteem shares significant variance in both mental well-being and happiness (Zimmerman, 2000). Self-esteem has been found to be the most dominant and powerful predictor of happiness (Furnham and Cheng, 2000). Indeed, while low self-esteem leads to maladjustment, positive self-esteem, internal standards and aspirations actively seem to contribute to 'wellbeing' (Garmezy, 1984; Glick and Zigler, 1992)."

The article concludes in summary, "Therefore, self-esteem enhancement can serve as a key component in...prevention and health promotion. The design and implementation of mental health programs with self-esteem as one of the core variables is an important and promising development in health promotion."

The benefits to self-esteem gained through a walking regimen can be immense, and in fact can be the greatest "take away" from such a program. This is the reason you find me encouraging you take full personal responsibility for every aspect of your walking program, and my recommendation that you walk at times alone when it is safe to do so. Walking is something we do for ourselves; it's personal. I want us to be clear, as we begin to like more and more the person we see in the mirror, feel more energetic, and become more likely to avoid self-defeating behaviors, we really only have one person to credit for these changes, ourselves. If low-self esteem is a downward spiral where one repeats the pattern of engaging in self-neglect, feeling additional low self-esteem because of it, then medicating that low self-esteem with more self-destructive and neglectful behavior, then we will not only stop that terrible cycle but turn it upside down. We will begin the formation of an upward spiral, one in which we like the person we are becoming more each day, step by step, walk by walk, and one where we suddenly start to seek-out more positive personal behaviors, in our diet, our relationships, in our modeling behavior for others and for ourselves. I can tell you there is something very beautiful which lies just ahead in your future. You will soon be able to reach out and touch it, like reaching out to touch the face you see reflected in the mirror, the one which once looked forlorn and fatigued but now perks up the corners of its lips and returns our gaze with a smile.

CHAPTER 17

TAKING OUR MINDS
FOR A WALK

As we saw in the last chapter, walking and other forms of exercise have a positive effect not only our physical health but our mental health as well, for we cannot escape the conspicuous truth that there is a deep symbiosis between our bodies and our minds. Not only do diet, personal habits, lifestyle, and activity level impact our overall health but our mind set does as well. So, if that is true, does what we think as we walk effect the health benefits of walking? The answer is a resounding yes. Imagine if we were going for a relaxing walk to enjoy some precious alone time then used that time to obsess about our personal problems. Here, in the act of walking, we are doing something beneficial for our general health then undermining it with negative thoughts. We need to work to keep our walking a positive experience both in our efforts to improve our physical health and mental health as well. Walking in both its physical and mental aspects should be a contrast to the stress-producing, health-depriving inputs of much of our daily life. Thoughts which are stress producing, self-esteem sabotaging, and generally depressing are the last things we want in our minds as we do something as beneficial and life-affirming as walking. So how do we control our thoughts as we walk and achieve some inner peace along the way? Here are some ideas.

In the beginning rather than immediately jumping fully into the more advanced positive thought techniques we are about to discuss, we must make sure we first learn to simply keep a positive attitude when we walk. For a time, this will be challenge enough. We want to encourage any positive thoughts we are having to continue, look around at the beautiful world in which we walk, and think about how we are benefiting by being out in the fresh air and truly living. We want to realize the significance of what we are doing, after all we are taking responsibility for our physical and mental health and we are taking the first steps in a life-changing journey. Let's just feel our bodies moving, feel them touching the earth, feel our muscles stretching and contracting, and embrace how good it feels. If outside worries start to enter our head, we will stop them, then switch back to more positive modes of thinking. In the beginning this is enough and a great accomplishment once we learn to do it consistently.

When we have difficulty keeping negative thoughts out of our heads there are really just two ways to eradicate them as we walk. One is to learn to let them go, simply ignoring them and allowing our brains to shift to more positive thoughts, or, secondly, to focus on something so intently that there is no room for negative thoughts to arise. But before we try either of these techniques I would suggest that first we start by getting to know the habits of our own mind. In our initial walks we need to get to know how our minds work and begin to develop our inner witness who sits back and watches the train of thoughts chugging through our very own brains. This new inner self is not the noisy monkey voice continually chatting inside our head, the one we listen to all day long, but the viewer who sits back and witnesses that voice and strives to keep it positive. Appendix 1 at the back of this book is titled Record Keeping. In the section of this appendix called *Walking Mind* we will learn how to keep a simple record of what goes on inside our brains as we walk. Most people find themselves thinking about a variety of things from the trivial to the meaningful, and which include both the good and the less good, the joyful and inspiring as well as the worrisome and negative. We will record what we discover as we begin to watch the habits of our own brains. Do we really have any control over what we think, or do our minds have a mind of their own?

If we allow our brains to randomly follow their own interests we will find that they spend a great deal of time hashing through material which generates concern, anxiety, stress, and doubt. While these are things we need to address to some degree in our lives, our health walks are not the time or place to do it. At that time our focus is on something different; we are interested in that which heals, on the positive and affirming and not those things which drag us down. Our walks create a kind of sacred ground where we choose to walk toward freedom and away from the confinement of our daily routines and liberate ourselves from mental stressors. We will need to learn how to protect this time and space, setting boundaries even for our own thinking. Remember the *Deep Walking* mantra taken from Dr. William Stewart's book *Deep Medicine* and repeat it often. "Everything we do and everything we think is either health affirming or health negating." On a daily basis I recommend that we begin to question ourselves about more of our actions and thoughts. Are they helping or hurting our progress toward better health? It's an important question. We must be sure to supply the answers as openly and honestly as we can.

Letting Go of Negative Thoughts

As I suggested earlier, one way to rid ourselves of the health-negating thoughts inside our head is to simply let them slide out of consciousness. For our thoughts to exist and to continue to exist once they form they need an accomplice, us. I am referring to us, the inner "viewers" and witnesses now, not us the ever-present thinkers, the ego providing persistent mind chatter. There are really two different entities inside our heads, we the "viewers" and inner witnesses and we the endlessly talking "drunken monkeys." If we the "viewers" don't participate in a monkey thought by holding it in focus, the thought will disappear and a new thought will form. Then when we do experience the development of a positive thought, as the "viewer" who determines what stays in our heads or leaves, we hold on to it. It is extremely important that when a negative thought enters our heads that we do not focus on it, either by encouraging it to continue or by trying to force it to leave. Attempting to force it out often makes it harder for it to go. The same dynamic exists in meditation, the type which attempts to free the mind of all forms of thought. When any thought enters, we must not empower it by resisting it, we must simply let it float away in the way that most thoughts do. If allowed to do so, thoughts evaporate as quickly and easily as they appear, like a raindrop on a hot summer sidewalk, but if we focus on them they endure like winter ice, covering our walking path and threaten to bring us down.

I do not expect for us to be able to do the following mental exercises throughout the duration of our walk. Perhaps at some point we will be able to gain that level of control over our ego mind's incessant activity. That does not apply to negative thinking which I hope we will quickly learn to avoid focusing on as we walk and at some point eradicate completely. However the following activities must be worked on slowly over time, and we will most likely be successful at first only for short periods of time. I assure you though it does get easier and the length of time we spend in these mind states will lengthen with practice. I remember how at first I thought of it as a kind of game. I would look ahead on my walking path to a turn in the trail up ahead or a specific bush or tree in the near distance and try to keep my mental focus until I arrived there. Over time the length of time I could stay in these states grew gradually and consistently.The letting negative thoughts float away approach takes some practice. We will record in our walking journals how it works for us.

Affirmations

Our second technique for keeping negative thoughts from forming is for some easier than the first and is accomplished by filling our heads with positive thoughts so there is no room for negative ones to form. One way this is done is through the use of affirmations. I will suggest some affirmations but it is really best to make-up our own. As we walk we will realize that one of the sounds which is most prevalent is the sound of our feet hitting the ground, so we will try to make our affirmations fit the beat and rhythm of our footfall. We must keep our affirmations relatively short in the beginning as the pace of our walking steps is initially slower. They can be of either an odd or even number of words. Simple three beat phrases like, "I feel good," or "Be here now," or "I am blessed," work well, but I find it best for mental focus to place a word between each phrase, a kind of silent step. "I feel good, yes...I feel good, yes....I feel good..." "I am alive and well, (step)...I am alive and well, (step)...I am alive and well..." The possibilities here are endless. Get creative.

"Finally it is time for me...Finally it is time for me..."

"I am free and filled with light...I am free and filled with light..."

"I feel strong, yes...I feel strong, yes...I feel strong, yes..."

"I am here and in the mo-ment...I am here and in the mo-ment..."

"Beauty all around me...beauty all around me..."

"Thank you for this gift...Thank you for this gift..."

"The time for me is now.."

"Love is in the moment...love is in the now...love is in the moment...love is in the now."

Affirmations not only help us to stay away from negative thinking, they keep our minds from wandering. Most importantly, however, they plant subconscious seeds of optimism within. The other night I watched the movie, *The Secret Garden*. Perhaps you have seen it. It is the story of two young cousins, one suffering from the emotional abandonment of her parents, the other succumbing to psychosomatic illness due to the loss of his mother and his father's subsequent depression and isolation. The boy's illness is so serious he is paralyzed with anxiety and fear to the extent he cannot walk, but the children soon discover a closed-off garden area on the estate in which they live and with the aid of a wheelchair for the boy sneak off to play there every day. They refer to it as their "secret garden," a place filled with birds and flowers, optimism and "magic" where they, through gardening, promote the health and growth of other living things, and thereby nurture and heal themselves. In the end the young emotionally paralyzed boy begins once again to walk. How appropriate.

This lovely little film helped me to understand that walking for me was my "secret garden," a place where I went each day to eradicate weeds and to plant the seeds of health within myself. Keeping negative thoughts out of our walking is like keeping noxious weeds away, and planting seeds of beautiful flowers is a lot like planting affirmations deep within the fertile ground inside ourselves. As we walk, we are in fact, not only doing something beneficial for ourselves today, we are tilling the earth and starting a beautiful garden which will flower and give us endless joy in the days which lie ahead.

Focusing on the Senses

The secret garden is an apt metaphor for our walks. It is a place which lies inside of us as much as outside of us, a place of peace and escape from the worries of the day, a place to heal and grow stronger, a counterbalance to the frenzy which tires us and wears us out, aging us well before our time. If you are fortunate as I am to have walking areas close by which are in beautiful natural settings then like me you often get to walk in an area that looks and feels like a real garden. If so, your walks are filled with sights and sounds, smells, tastes and tactile impressions which are naturally attractive and which have the power to draw you into positive feelings and distract you away from any missteps toward negative thoughts and attitudes. How does one think of the dirty laundry back home which needs to be done when they are surrounded by flowers and bird song? We can use these powerful attractors in the natural world around us as sensual affirmations. This "Beauty-all-around-me-work" as I call it will help us develop greater mindfulness and enhance our focusing skills as we learn to "be here now" rather than ruminating about the past or worrying about the future. It will also help us focus more on being grateful for what we have rather than focusing on what is lacking. Living more fully in the moment and being grateful for the miracle which is our lives are two of the keys to good mental health and happiness. I often find myself reciting the Native American poem, "Beauty before me, beauty behind me, beauty above me, beauty below me, beauty all around me, I walk in beauty."

When we are walking and find ourselves drawn to one of the natural world's beautiful attractors in our immediate environment we need to try to eradicate all thinking and focus only on the sensual experience itself. Perhaps it is a smell in the air, the sound of the wind in the trees, a wildflower along the path. Perhaps we are drawn to the sound of our own breathing or the sound of our feet hitting the earth. Let's focus on that. Let's see how long we can keep any form of internal monologue silent as we focus on the external world. Yielding control for a moment in the moment, we stop analyzing and continually transforming the world around us into words which then run wildly through our heads. We get to that place which is bigger than language, more inclusive than words and go with it, seeing how long we can keep focused on some simple beautiful sense experience without needing to deflate it by reducing it to the reductive symbols of language.

There is an old Zen story of two great monks who when they first met went to sit together in a lovely garden. They sat there together for a long time without either of them speaking. Finally one them turned to the other and said, "They call that thing over there a tree." They both began to chuckle and then doubled up with laughter. The joke, of course, was that both understood that the labels we place on objects in the world in no way represent the phenomenal reality they truly are. In fact our constant mental cataloging of all the individual components of the life miracle in part destroys it, and can even assist in the development of a hurtful mental belief: that the wondrous world around us is a collection of individual parts rather than the unified whole it really is. In truth we are not separated from it any more than we are separated from our bodies, and knowing this allows us to use the power of the whole both in body and in nature to promote the health of each of us as the separate individuals we imagine ourselves to be.

If we "think" during these encounters at all, we need to think about how the words in our heads often separate us from our own feelings and from a deeper connection to the biological world. Think about how that separation is a form of illness itself and a cause of illnesses for mind and body many of us fall victim to. Think about what we can do to break down the wall between our mind and body, between our thoughts and the natural world and use that renewed connection for greater health. Be mindful, be present, be grateful. We are after all walking now on a new path which is leading to the birth of someone new. That someone is the new person we are creating. We are heading to a place beyond simple physical fitness to fitness of body, mind, and spirit. I get excited just thinking about where this path will lead us, and it gives me joy. One day very soon, if not already, you will begin to understand why.

When we are ready, when we are walking regularly and able to focus with a positive mindset while walking we need to try some of the mental exercises above. Try them all. They get easier over time. Try one for a while and then another. You will be surprised at how quickly they become second nature during your walking outings, and you will be even more surprised at how they will benefit your life when you are not walking at all.

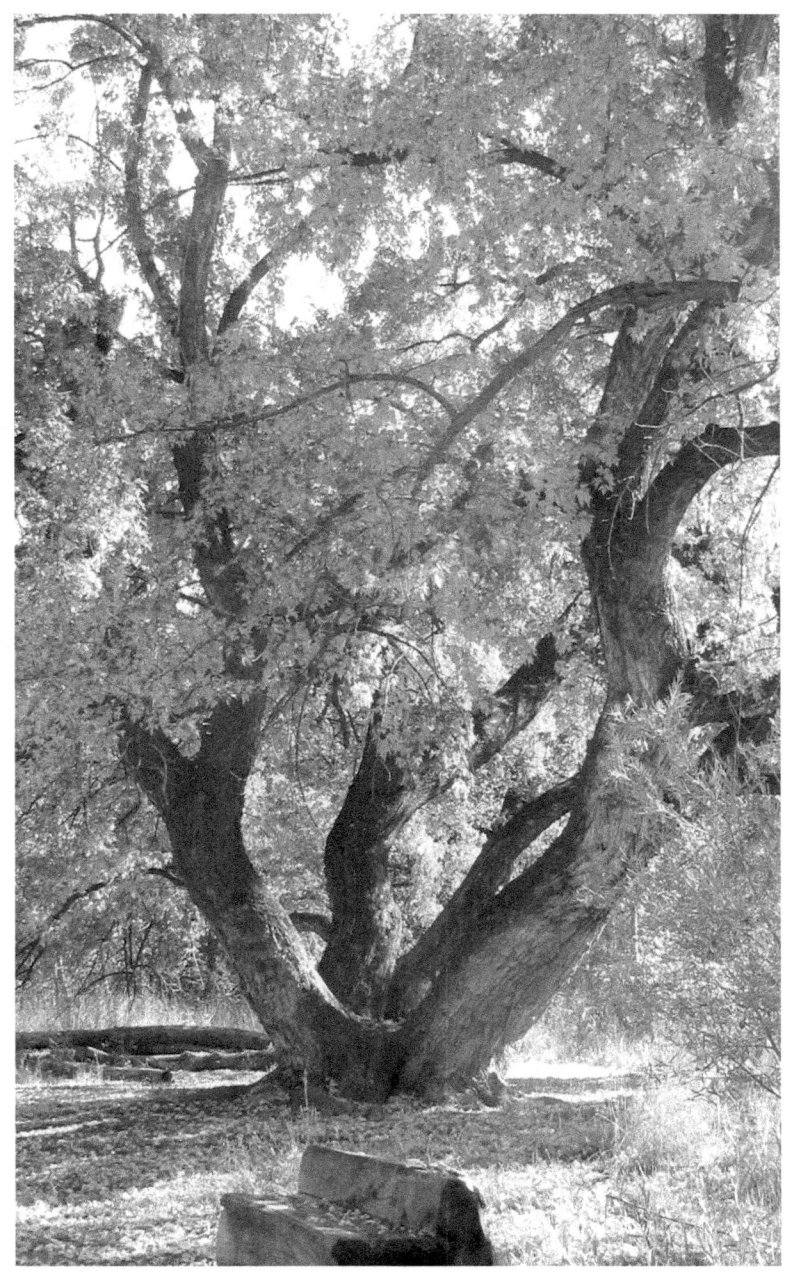

CHAPTER 18

THE BENEFITS OF MEDITATION

More and more people in both the professional and lay communities are recognizing the importance of taking time to quiet the mind. The rapid and stressful pace of our lives makes it something not just desirable to change but absolutely necessary. For our general health we must learn not only to exercise the body but to rest the brain, for very few of us have to worry about having an under-exercised mind. It is after all one organ of the body which gets a continuous workout, so much so it risks being overworked and burnt-out. If the mind's daily workout only included substantive reading and challenging problem solving punctuated with moments of peace, contemplation, and joy then there would be little concern, but for the majority of us our brain's workout is primarily filled with senseless worry, negative thinking, and continual distractions. These things are not only non-nutritious from the point-of-view of mental health, but are in many ways toxic. It is the mind's form of junk food and a diet which in the long run can damage both mind and body.

Meditation, a practice of calming, focusing and quieting the mind has existed in many cultures for thousands of years. What once was seen as the mysterious and unusual activities of Eastern Yogis has long ago become mainstream in much of our own Western culture. A 2007 study by the U.S. government found that over 20 million adults had practiced meditation in the past 12 months. The truth is, meditation has been an important activity for thousands of years in the Western World as well as the Eastern World. In both the East and West, meditation has been associated with spiritual training and can be found in some form in Christianity, Islam, Buddhism and Hinduism. While we most often associate meditation with Eastern religious traditions, meditation also has a long history in Christianity. Christian meditation is, however, centered more on Biblical text than on developing mindfulness or generating states of inner emptiness, its primary goal being to develop a closer relationship with God by contemplating the many aspects of His word. In contrast, among Christian mystics, meditative techniques have been used largely to establish a direct connection with God, with a primary emphasis on ecstatic experience. In the East, meditation has been used not only to contemplate the godhead as Chiristians often use it, but to quiet the mind and to focus on emptiness as a way to cleanse the mind and enrich one's perception of the world.

In the 20th and 21st centuries, however, meditation has taken a more practical turn and become popular in secular society and the subject of scientific inquiry. Those studies have come to some interesting conclusions. It has been found that a few minutes a day of inner reflection and quieting of mind with a focus on the present moment can highly reduce stress and facilitate our daily decision making. We are learning that this decrease in stress resulting from meditation activities is also seen in numerous studies to decrease the possibility of heart disease and many other stress related illnesses, and learning also that stress is in fact a determinant factor in the development of nearly all illnesses.

Through meditation techniques we can learn to control our thoughts. How is this beneficial? The answer is that by being able to control and stop distracting thoughts which side-track our thinking, by teaching us how to keep negative thinking from undermining our positive attitude, and by showing us that our lives are in large part the things we focus on in our heads, we can change the focus of our thoughts and thereby change our lives. Meditation is a form of mental conditioning which can actually provide a form of mental fitness which helps whip an unruly and unfit mind into shape, and a fit mind goes a very long way in terms of helping us achieve our desired goals in a walking regimen or in life in general, just as an unfit mind makes it far more difficult to do so.

Meditation can also help us develop a form of healthy detachment from the endless list of little things which irritate us during the day. I am sure you have seen how the mind can turn a small setback into a great trauma in no time at all. "I have missed one day of walking, so I might as well give up." Or someone cuts us off in traffic; we slow down to avoid a collision and then we start to boil. Soon this person who has cut us off, who at first was just an inconsiderate boob driven by self-interest becomes with the assistance of mind a threat to the very existence of the free world, a danger to the well-being of all. I think of this as the "mind as magnifying glass syndrome" and it has been at the center of many a road-rage incident. Meditation helps us see things without magnification, be they fears, insults, slights, worries and various other routine agitations. Wouldn't it be nice to have a little more stability and rather than letting small things throw us for a loop be able to keep our cool as we assess a problem and see it in a clear perspective, taking real problems head-on but not sweating disproportionately the small stuff?

Where does happiness come from? Does it come from the sources outside of ourselves, from the things and people with whom we associate or does it come from within, from something we call peace of mind? The truth is that no matter how much we gain from the outside world, be they material possessions, jobs, or valued relationships, they mean little unless we are happy within ourselves. If we have peace of mind we feel happy, and if we feel happy we have better mental health, and if we have mental health we are naturally inclined to move toward improved physical health. And the opposite is true, people who are inactive, overweight, unfit, and in general live an unhealthy lifestyle often do so because they are at core unhappy. Meditation helps us find greater happiness by teaching us that happiness is not dependent on outer circumstances, and by giving us the tools to find happiness within.

We live more and more in a world of constant distraction. Be it the busyness of our personal lives or the flickering consciousness promoted in part by computers, television, and smart phones, we are losing our ability to concentrate on anything for any extended period of time. In his book, *The Shallows: What the Internet is Doing to Our Brains*, Nicholas Carr suggests we are becoming "pancake people," people whose knowledge and focus is wide but extremely thin. Not only are we losing our capacity for deep thinking and awareness, giving up insight and wisdom for a superficial knowledge of meaningless facts, we are also losing our ability to concentrate and focus, which is a problem because we need focus and deep concentration to achieve our human potential. Meditation is largely based on teaching us how to focus mindfully on one thing at a time, thereby giving us new skills of concentration which we can carry into our daily lives and help us achieve the life goals we desire.

Much of the monkey mental chatter which fills our heads each day and which we mistakenly think of as our inner self when in truth it is just our chatty ego, deals with things that have already happened or things we anticipate may happen. Research indicates that 90% of our mental worry does us no good. In other words, the majority of what goes on inside of our heads is about the past and future and has little to do with the present, the here and now, the only time and place where we can really do much about anything. If we live in our heads and listen only to the ranting monkey he will steal our lives, dragging us into what is gone or what might come and keeping us away from the moment, the very place where life is lived. The current moment is the home of creativity and spontaneous being. It is also the place where happiness and joyousness resides.

Again, one of principal objectives of meditation is to help us quiet monkey mind and to free us from obsessing about the past and future and to teach us how to live in the moment. These are meditation's greatest gifts. As you begin to do some of the mental exercises in this book don't be surprised if your life starts to take a turn toward the spontaneous and creative, or you find yourself spending more time in the now. For here too is the home of our true selves, someone we can get to know once we learn how to enter the deep insightful silence and convince the monkey-ego to hold his tongue, at least long enough for us to hear a new and powerful voice which is being born and rising up within.

Meditation takes two basic forms, at least here in the Western world. They are concentrative meditation and mindful meditation. Concentrative meditation uses a focused attention on a specific thought, sight, sound, or feeling, while mindful meditation is a kind of close and focused monitoring of what we are experiencing in our daily actions and thoughts. Concentrative meditation requires the voluntary focus on a single object, word or thought, and mindful meditation stands back and watches the detailed unfolding of our actions and thoughts or the moment to moment ebb and flow of our sensory experiences. Our use of affirmations is a form of concentrative meditation, and watching our thoughts and letting the negative ones slip away is a form of mindful meditation. Focusing on the sound of our footsteps as we walk is concentrative meditation, focusing on our feet stepping over the earth as it unfolds before us in a string of moment by moment particulars, mindful meditation.

One helpful way to think of meditation in general is to think of it as starting a campfire. We need fuel, air, and fire in order to start one. The fuel is our physical brain, the air the thoughts contained therein, and the fire our mental focus whether we are concentrating on one thing or monitoring with our "inner witness" a series of actions or thoughts. The purpose of our campfire is to create a light so that we can see better in the dark, but to do this, we must keep the fire burning consistently and brightly. As we meditate, our focus, particularly in the beginning, will fluctuate. We will slip in and out of focus as our concentration alternates between burning brightly and then fades back to glowing coals.

Our goal is to get to a point where we can keep the fire burning brightly. This happens only with practice, but even the early lower light flickering flame meditations are extremely beneficial, and important steps along the way.

In our use of walking meditation we will use the mindfulness technique primarily. We will have already staked out our "secret garden" as a place where negative thinking is not allowed, and learned to let negative thoughts just "float away". And we will also have planted seeds by concentrating on positive affirmations, and done more concentrated meditation by visually focusing on objects in our view as we walked, or by focusing on repetitious sounds like our footsteps or our breathing. These are wonderful ways to prepare the ground, to collect the fuel and start the campfire burning. Now through mindful walking meditation we will turn the little fire we have ignited into a raging blaze. Fire is an amazing thing. Have you ever thought about how incredible it is that a single match with its small little flame can easily become a massive forest fire?

CHAPTER 19

WALKING MEDITATION

First Meditation: Thought focusing

For our first attempt at walking meditation, let's start by thinking of only one word as we walk. For instance, each time our right foot hits the ground let's think to ourselves, "step." When our left foot touches down think of nothing or of silence. In our mind we will hear only this, "step(silence), step(silence), step(silence), step." If we find other thoughts trying to work their way into our step and silence thoughts, refocus, let the intrusive thoughts slip away and return once again to only this pattern, "step(silence), step(silence), step(silence)..." We want to do this until we can go some distance without thinking of anything other than the repetition of "step(silence), step(silence)." Remember our campfire analogy. When the only thing in our mind is the word step surrounded by empty silence the campfire gets brighter; when an external thought enters or something in our field of senses grabs our attention, the campfire fades. In the beginning we don't want to try to do this exercise for the full duration of our walk. Just use it off and on until it gets easier, the length of our concentration becomes longer, and our campfire burns brighter.

Second Meditation: Slowing down the mind.

In the fast pace of our daily lives our minds become habituated to rapid thinking and covering a diverse variety of topics over a short period of time. This is a good skill to have with our current hyper-busy multi-tasking lifestyles but comes with a great cost. That cost is ultimately our loss of the ability to achieve deep focus, sharp concentration, and the loss of the ability to live in the moment rather than living in the past or future. We miss so much of life because our minds are used to quickly moving on to the next interest, often times before it has time to understand and digest the last interest. Not only do we spend too much time living inside of our heads to the exclusion of other ways of experiencing the world, when lost in head thought we are constantly distracted and moving on to whatever the next thought happens to be. We are often attracted to a thought then distracted by the next thought before we have fully comprehended the first thought. To help combat this problem during out walking regimen we need to make the mind more mindful of every passing moment, and keep it focused on a single thought or action. Here is how we do it.

Once we have worked on the "step(silence), step," exercise we need to add a little more complexity to the words inside our head. Say now "left, right, left, right," as each foot hits the ground and without silence in between. See how far you can walk without any other words than "left" and "right" entering your mind. If other word thoughts start to enter refocus only on "left" and "right." Work on this meditation for at least a portion of the time on your future walks until you can go some distance with only the words "left" and "right" going through your mind. When we get comfortable with this, we will add even more details of each footstep to occupy our mind more fully. Now, rather than just being mindful of each step, we will try to become more mindful of smaller facets of each step. We may have to slow our walking pace down in order to do this because we are thinking of more words in the same amount of time. Next, let's try to focus even more on what our leg and foot are doing with each step. Do it with only one leg at a time; say, "lifting, setting down" (silence as your other leg is moving), "lifting, setting down" (silence as the other leg moves) "lifting, setting down." Try this for a while and see how well you do. The goal of this type of mindful meditation can continue to progress to what ever degree we are capable of. Eventually we can try to get to a point where we can be mindful of up to four phases of movement in the stride of each leg. Again, focusing on one leg at a time. Then we will be thinking to ourselves "lift, stepping forward, stepping down, touching ground (silence as the other leg moves) then "lift, stepping forward, stepping down, touching ground" again. So we won't have to slow our walking down too much to do this, we not only think of the movement of just one leg as it goes through these motions, we empty our minds completely as the second leg goes through the same movements. When we have successfully done this we switch to the other leg, then back again. Don't try to do all of the first and second meditations above during one walk. At least at first. Work on one of these meditations over a number of walks until you get it down then move on to the next one.

We can do this type of mindful exercise for any movement of our body. Let's try being mindful of each phase of our breathing, "filling up, letting go, filling up, letting go." We can focus on our arm movement as well, "swinging back, moving forward, swinging back." Again, it will be a bit difficult to have thoughts containing this many words in the time it takes our body to complete the movement we describe, so limit it to the movement of one arm at a time or slow your pace way down or use less words in the description of the movement. As we get better at these mindfulness activities we will see how long we can walk with just the mindful thoughts of movement in our head and without any other thoughts intervening. Once again let's try to make it to a tree, a telephone pole, or a turn in the path we see up ahead while being totally mindful. In Appendix 1, Keeping a Record, there is a section devoted to recording the effects you experience while doing these mind exercises. Be sure to jot down a few thoughts about your mindful activity experiences there.

After doing mindful exercises for a time, we will learn some very interesting things, not the least of which is that we can actually train our mind to focus on something for an extended period of time. This will make us more conscious of the wandering focus typical of our mind in daily life, teaching us that our mind usually works in a way which is quite arbitrary and scattered and can be the first step in gaining control of our thinking and learning to think more deeply and mindfully even during times when we are not walking at all.

One of the most important things Eastern yogis learn from mindfulness activities is that body and mind are inseparably linked just as we have noted in our discussion of the integration of mental and physical health and our goal of healing the mind/body split. For every movement of the body there is a corresponding awareness of mind. Often times this awareness is subliminal, but never-the-less the mind at some level is aware of the body whether or not we are consciously aware of it or not. In the far East the term Nama is used for the mind, while the name for things of the material world are Rupa, or matter. Nama and Rupa are interwoven into a unified fabric which shares an interesting commonality: they both can arise and disappear within a single moment. This perpetual coming and going of both the physical and mental, this lack of permanence as thoughts and things arise out of nothing and return to nothing in the end corroborates the Eastern philosophical belief that all things arise out of the ground being of nothingness and returns to that ground when they pass. All things be they Nama or Rupa are born of the silent void which surrounds them and return to that void when they are done. It is important to remember that the void in many Eastern traditions is different than our conception of it here in the West. It is not so much the absence of everything, a vast and empty nothingness, but the presence of everything, a kind of source ground or "luminous emptiness" which contains all potential actions, objects, and thoughts. In much the same way as white light contains all colors of the spectrum the void contains all the colors of possibility and potentiality. In this sense, emptiness, silence, and absence are seen as the well-spring for all that comes into being and the place to which it all returns, at all levels, be it thoughts and physical actions or the coming and going of individual lives.

This view of ultimate reality which once seemed strange to Westerners, is now becoming a commonplace explanation for phenomena since the development of the "New Physics" over the last one hundred years. The new laws of quantum mechanics reflect the understanding that our material reality at the atomic level is 99% emptiness and 1% matter. There are vast quantities of space between every tiny particle of matter, and this is as true for the human body at that level as it is for the universe as a whole. When it was discovered that things were composed of 99% emptiness in the early part of the twentieth century one physicist noted that he was afraid to get out of bed in the morning for fear of falling through his bedroom floor. The new physics is also teaching us that what we once thought of as nothingness, empty space, the void, is actually filled with other forms of matter and energy we cannot see. They are known in physics today as dark energy and dark matter. It is these invisible forms of matter and energy which constitute 95% of the universe in which we live yet we can't see and which could, as some speculate, be ultimately the source ground for everything our senses detect in the world.

Quantum mechanics also teaches us that much of what we see at the microscopic level does not follow rules of hard certainty like the rules operative in the world we know. Instead it follows rules of probability based to an extent upon the way an observer views them. The new physics is teaching us that foundational reality, the one we find at the subatomic level, is in a state of constant flux and uncertainty, and which from the observer's viewpoint moves continually in and out of being and manifests itself in many possible forms and in many times and places. There is a perpetual dance between matter and the void, much like the interplay of the human mind and the material world. The world we know exists as it does because of it, and provides the basic dynamic of our lives: coming into being, returning to the void, coming from the void, entering into being. It seems that at all levels our existence may be created by the interaction of Nama and Rupa.

It would be easy to dispel the theories of the New Physics and write them off as far-out hypothetical theories if it wasn't for the fact that they have been proven in the scientific laboratory and corroborated by numerous experiments over the last 100 years and have helped form the foundation for all of the digital technology we currently enjoy. In fact, Steven Hawking maintains that the theories of quantum mechanics are the most tested and validated theories in the history of science.

Another important concept we discover as we mindfully meditate is that Nama (mind) precedes the movement of Rupa (matter). We must desire to move our legs when we walk and, until we convert that desire into mental "intent" and focus, nothing moves. We get little accomplished when we simply want to do something, for wanting alone doesn't get things done. We still have to convert want into willful mental intent and when we do so our legs begin to lift, move forward, step down then touch the ground. This fact is obvious when we slow down our walking and become mindful of every movement. The mind must focus on the idea that I want my legs to move before they are able to do so. But this simple understanding has some larger implications: it reveals not only the connection and interdependence of our bodies and minds but also teaches us about the power of intent. You may have always wanted to read a book about walking but you never "intended" to pick one up and read it. If you had you would have already read one. You may have had a burning desire to start a serious walking regimen but because you never went on to the stage of converting that desire into mental intent you continued to sit and nothing moved. All the wonderful thoughts about possible actions remain only in our heads and fail to manifest in the material world if there is no intent to make them do so. We must have the thought that we want to walk then have the intent to begin our walk before we walk at all.

What we are ultimately talking about here is the amazing power of the mind to get things done and the recognition that without the intentional power of mind nothing does get done. Again that seems obvious, but why then do millions of people every day with wonderful ideas percolating in their heads stop short and never truly "intend" something into being. Do they just not know that wanting something to happen is not by itself enough? Why do people want to exercise and do not exercise, why do some people want to get out of a bad relationship or job but never do? It's because they lack the power of willful intent.

The truth is that without intent nothing changes, just as it is true that with intent even the smallest ant can build a giant mountain (at least by ant standards). By understanding the true power of intent we have the ability to change our lives when change is needed. Intent moves our feet as we walk down a trail, intent moves us out of a bad situation, intent builds pyramids and great civilizations and even takes humans to the moon. Wanting alone has never done that. I hope that by doing some mindful meditation exercise we will all come to understand the power of our thoughts. Most of the changes that have occurred throughout history started with a simple thought (Nama) which was changed into action or matter (Rupa) with intent. When we begin to use our own powerful intent to establish and continue a life-long walking routine our desires will at last begin to manifest.

When we walk we should never take it for granted, seeing it as just a little something we do for our health. Think of it instead as a form of personal empowerment. "I intended to walk and now I am walking." "I intended to walk on a regular basis and now I am doing so." You will find that the lessons we learn in the simple act of mindful walking can have truly dramatic effects when we begin to apply them to other aspects of our lives. "I always wanted to have a better job but not until I intended to have a better job did I have one." If you realize the true power of intent and use it, you can accomplish whatever you choose. I can attest to this myself. I wanted to write a book about walking for some time, but until I coupled that desire with concentrated intent no words magically showed up on the page. As you can see I finally achieved it; I finally got to the stage of not just wishing a book would appear but of mentally telling my fingers to move across the keys of my word processor just as I had willed my legs to rise and fall as I walked down my walking path. Now the book has appeared to manifest right before my eyes. But let's move on now, for I intend to write a short paragraph about impermanence. Let's see if my intent is strong enough to do so.

We talked briefly above about the way we discover through walking meditation how thoughts seem to originate from nothing and create a movement in the world which itself ultimately disappears and is replaced by a new thought intention which arises and creates more motion. Not only do we learn through the great silence which surrounds us and the vast emptiness of inner and outer space from which thoughts and movement come into being, we also learn about the laws of impermanence. Thoughts, things, people, events, everything seems to come into being then in time goes back to the void. For many of us this a frightening thought. We have a natural longing for permanence and the security and stability it affords. Still, permanence is ultimately the greatest illusion; things may appear to remain constant and not disappear but this is only an illusion created by our limited perspective. The earth seems unchanging until we look at how it has changed geologically from the perspective of millions of years.

"But it will continue to exist forever in some form won't it?" I can hear someone out there asking. No, it came into being and one day it will go out of being like everything else. We don't like to think about this element of reality because we get attached to some things and do not want them to change. If we love someone we certainly do not want them to change in relation to us or to go out of being, and we will use our strongest intent to make sure that doesn't happen. We don't want our great job to end, or to lose the house we have worked so hard to own. Still, all of these things will one day pass regardless of how hard we try to hold on to them. It is a hard pill to swallow, but all the things and relationships we love so much will end and the earth will continue to spin on without us, but not forever, for one day it too will stop spinning. While it might at first make us sad to contemplate this reality of life, if we learn to accept it we can actually gain tremendous personal strength and understanding from it. How?

Living as though life will go on endlessly is a good way to miss its incredible though transient beauty and a precursor to lacking the gratitude needed to fully appreciate the gift it is. At a deep level all things in life are enhanced by the fact that they will not last forever, including life itself. By actually focusing on life's impermanence---something many people desire to avoid---we heighten the power and beauty of each moment and have greater gratitude for this great miracle which each of us enjoys. Seeing our thoughts and movements during walking meditation come and go, seeing each of them come from emptiness and return to emptiness makes us more aware not only of each thought and action but of the silent void from which they spring and into which they will return. What would music sound like if it was eternal, if it had no beginning or end and there was no silence between individual notes? It would undoubtedly sound like so much noise. As many great musicians have said from Miles Davis to B.B. King, the silence around musical notes is just as important as the notes which are sounded and these two artists in particular are known as much for the notes they did not play as for those they did. The silence which surrounds every individual thought and action in our lives is just as important and beautiful as the silence existent before we lived and the silence which will follow when we stop doing so, for ultimately without silence there is no sound just as without sound there's no such thing as silence.

While engaged in walking meditation we spend a lot of time being mindful of every detail of each thought and action and recognizing and accepting the fact of their impermanence. And I repeat, this makes us more mindful and appreciative of each detail in our lives and also helps us see the beauty of non-being, of the space and silence which surrounds us and in which we function and live. Also, when we pay greater attention to life's comings and goings and understand the inevitability of their passing we develop a different attitude toward them. While on one hand we appreciate them much more, on the other hand we attach to them a little less strongly. Through this we also learn that we do not have to completely attach to something to appreciate it or to enjoy it. In fact the opposite is true, we appreciate a gift more when we understand it will not last forever. The Western world's obsession with comfort, sameness, predictability, stability, and permanence is not only a self-generated delusion, impossible to achieve in the real world, but the ultimate life-stealer. What is stolen is the very richness of life itself. If we know that like our footsteps our relationships will come and go, our material possessions will come and go, our work and various life stages will come and go, and every year will come and go just as our very lives will come and go, our appreciation of what we have in the present moment will sky rocket out of sight.

When we talk about developing non-attachment through meditation, we are not talking about non-appreciation or under-valuing the people and things in our lives, just the opposite. We are talking about giving up the kind of attachment that wants things to stay the same and never change, the kind of attachment based in a fear of the new and a terror of the unknown. This kind of attach-ment is both unrealistic and undesirable, at least for those of us who want a deeper and more fulfilling life experience.

Let's be clear, walking meditation is actually a type of prac-tice, and what we are practicing is not only mind rest, non-negative thinking, focusing skills, and being present in the moment, but a way of practicing to see our lives more fully and thereby enabling us to live them more deeply. When we stop and truly pay atten-tion to something, slow it down and see its numerous facets and details because we know it will not last, we internalize it much more fully. In the rat race of our daily lives so much goes unno-ticed. The rat doesn't have time to stop and ponder, for while he has no idea where he is going he knows he needs to get there fast. But we wouldn't walk past a Van Gogh painting would we? We wouldn't go to the Metropolitan Museum without constantly stop-ping and taking time to examine its magnificent paintings in detail? Perhaps not. But we must remember something else which we will learn through meditative walking, every moment of the life we live is itself a beautiful painting, and if we do not take time to value it fully there is little reason to have come to the great museum of life in the first place.

More and more humans live in the world like water skippers carrying an Instacam. We live a life taking snapshots, a quick shot here and there to stick in a photo album we seldom take time to view. Unfortunately many of us have become used to skimming across the surface of life like water skippers across a pond, taking quick and easy pictures of the passing of our lives. Through meditation we are trying to become more like fish swimming throughout the pond, from side to side and top to bottom, fish which explore the water's breadth and depth and use an underwater movie camera to capture experiences so we don't miss a single frame of the beauty all around us. Here is the longer form of the famous anonymous Navaho prayer I paraphrased part of earlier:

"Today I will walk out, today everything negative will leave me.
I will be as I was before, I will have a cool breeze over my body.
I will have a light body, I will be happy forever, nothing will hinder me.
I walk with beauty before me. I walk with beauty behind me.
I walk with beauty below me. I walk with beauty above me.
I walk with beauty around me. My words will be beautiful.
In beauty all day long may I walk."

As you walk and practice your mindful meditations, the movie camera analogy is an excellent one to keep in mind. As the thought to lift your leg and move your foot forward enters your mind and you use your intent to make it move, see the movement first as two snapshots, one of your knee starting to lift, the second of your foot touching the ground. Even this is more mindful than we usually are. We normally would walk without thinking about our leg movement at all, focused possibly on some worry or concern of the day. So kudos to those of you who achieve even basic mindfulness, it is a big leap forward compared to the norm. Still, before we pat ourselves on our backs too much, remember that if we had used a movie camera to film our leg movement there would be hundreds of individual frames which showed minute yet different perspectives of our leg movement, and if we were mindful enough we would actually be aware of all these variations as we walked. It has been said that the Buddha was this mindful in every act he performed, from eating a meal to greeting someone he did not know. We all need to slow things down and be more present. Perhaps, as I have, you have known people who were so busy talking during dinner that afterwards they had forgotten what they had eaten, or met someone who when you first met them seemed totally focused on something else, leaving you feeling like you were invisible and unimportant, and if you are like me, you have been one of those people too.

Again we use mindful meditation in part to help keep our minds free from other thoughts, meaningless and sometimes hurtful thoughts which we avoid while we walk. This form of meditation also helps us focus on the subject at hand rather than letting the mind aimlessly wander wherever it will, and helps us learn to control our thinking too. We use it also to help us learn to be more present in the moment during our walks with the understanding that that skill will then be carried over into other parts of our day, for the time we reserve for meditative walking is not the only time we need to be mindful. My hope is that as we become more mindful it will eventually be applied to other parts of our lives and thereby enrich them. The following is an outline for a mindful walking event, but as you will see we could simply substitute a few new words into that outline and apply it to a vast number of other things we experience throughout our day.

Mindful Focus on Our Bodies as We Walk

1. After warming up stand still before starting your walk. Feel your feet where they meet the ground. Be aware of how all of your weight goes down your legs and through your feet. Notice the slight adjustments your body makes while simply standing upright in order not to fall.

2. Begin walking and focus on the way you walk. Is your stride long or short, are you moving at a slow or fast pace? Feel the muscles in your legs. Are they stiff or relaxed? What are your arms doing?

3. Now pay closer attention to your feet. Notice how your weight shifted through your feet from heel to toe and back again. Decipher the pattern of that movement and imagine it as it occurs over and over again.

4. Feel your ankles and lower legs now. Can you focus on your ankles and feel how they move? Is it mostly forward or side to side? Feel them relax as you start your walk. Notice how they move individually and as a part of your whole leg movement. Sense also your calves and shins. Can you focus so that you only feel that part of your body? How do your calf muscles work in relation to the rest of your legs and feet?

5. Move your awareness up to your thighs. Sense where your clothes comes in contact with them. Focus on the muscles of your thigh. Can you distinguish between those muscles in front and those in the back? Sense your hip joints? Is there any discomfort? Feel now your entire hip region. How does your hip move as your walk? Does one side lift as the other goes down?

6. How does your stomach feel? Walking actually strengthens the stomach muscles over time. Can you feel it?

7. Your chest is in constant movement too. Not only does it move as your arms swing back and forth but it rises and falls with your breathing. Can you feel that? Can you hear yourself breathe? Is it deep or shallow? Can you count your breaths, first by counting as you exhale then as you inhale too?

8. Pay attention to your shoulders now. Watch their rhythmic movement. Notice how they move opposite to your hips.

9. Focus now on your arms. Feel them in detail starting from you upper arms to forearms then your wrists and hands. How do your arms move? Do they simply hang down to your sides? Do they rise up in front of you as you walk? Pay now particular attention to your hands. Are your fingers open or closed? What does it feel like as your hands move through the air? How does it affect the way you feel?

10. Shift your focus to your neck area. The muscles in your neck support your head. How do those muscles feel? What does your head do as you walk? Does it move? If so, does it move forward and backward, side to side, or up and down?

11. Pay close attention now to your face. The face has hundreds of muscles. Feel your jaw. Is it relaxed or set? If it is tight, relax it. What are your eyes doing? Are they looking around or focusing straight ahead? Try for a time to just keep a general focus on what is ahead of you without focusing on one thing in particular. Scan upward until you reach the horizon line. What do your see peripherally still looking straight ahead but focusing for a moment on what you see passing quickly to the sides of you. Now focus once again to what lies in front of you.

12. When you end your walk and before you start your cool down stretching, stand still for just a moment and perceive what it feels like to stop and stand after walking. How does your body feel overall? What do your legs feel like after walking then simply standing? Feel how your weight once again is directly over your feet. Note how they feel and what it feels like to be once more anchored to the ground after spending time striding over the earth's surface. Focus on the contrast of movement and non-movement. Think about stillness followed by movement, followed by stillness. Think about being inactive then using your intent to move, then moving, then what it feels like afterwards. First there was stillness, then you had the idea of walking. You used your intent to go walking and now you have completed your walk and it has returned to the stillness from which it came. How does that feel? Take a minute just to appreciate what you have done. Experience yourself standing there at the end of your walk, experiencing what you feel in body and mind. Feel gratitude for being alive and being able to walk at all.

Mindful Sensual Focus on a Flower along the Path

1. As you walk, try to find a flower growing along your path. Try to see the flower as if you are seeing a flower for the first time, like a child or an alien from another planet. What is it that made you stop? Something obviously attracted you, what was it?

2. Was it the flower's color? Focus for a moment just on its color. What is it about this color you find appealing? Is the color bright or subdued? What does the color make you feel?

3. Look at the flower's shape. How many petals does it have? Do you find the flower's shape attractive? Can you associate any kind of feeling the shape of the flower inspires in you? Which attracts you most, the flower's color or shape? Perhaps it is the combination of the two. What is it about the shape you like?

4. Bend over and smell the flower. What does it smell like? Is it a pleasant smell or non-descript? Is it subtle or strong? Have you smelled something like this before or is it a smell unlike any other you have smelled? Does the smell make the flower more attractive to you or less so?

5. When you touch the flower petals are they soft or hard? Do they feel the way you expected them to? How about the stem? Does it feel rough, does it have thorns? Would you call this flower delicate or hardy? Perhaps it is both.

6. Put your face close to the flower. How does this change what you experience and feel or think? Does your closeness or distance make a difference in what you see or what you feel?

7. Step back now and look at the flower from a distance. Does it look any different now than it did when you first came upon it. Compare both perspectives, what you felt when you first came upon the flower and now how you feel about it after looking at it mindfully.

8. As you stand now and look at the flower think about what is happening. You are on a walk and came across something that drew you to it. You took a moment to appreciate it and to look it over in greater detail. You and the flower are separate but share life and a place on the walking path. For a moment you stopped for a mindful exploration of something you may have come to take for granted. Having stopped, how do you feel about the flower now? Has it enhanced your attraction to it? Had you ever looked this closely at a flower before?

9. As you stand before the flower think about what appears to be the distance between you. We often see ourselves as separate, outside of the things we observe in the world, and even the things we share life with. What is it which makes us feel so separate from the people and things we share the gift of living with? Did you feel the wall of separateness between you and the flower break down when you did your best to really see it?

10. Before you continue your walk and turn your back to the flower which first attracted you and inspired your attention, think for a moment about how a flower on your walking path is like all of the people, objects and events you experience on your walk down life's path. How can you affect how you feel about those things by taking time to appreciate them and by experiencing them more fully and mindfully? How can you break down the

wall of separation largely created by the human ego? How can you share a deeper connection and communion, a mutual love and respect for all the other things you share life with?

We will want to work on our mindfulness training a little each time we walk. How many different things are there available to be mindful of? The answer is that there are an infinite number. There is literally no limit to the things we can see, smell, touch, feel and hear as we walk. What would happen if we began to look at them all with a little more mindfulness? And what would happen if by being more mindful when we went walking it made it easier for us to be more mindful all the time? We should ask ourselves one important question. How would a child, a friend, a pet, a home, a marriage, a possession, a family, or anything else look to us if we became capable of appreciating them with a greater depth and richness? How would these things be transformed if we gave mindful focus to each, rather than viewing them like things we see peripherally as we walk, an image slightly out of focus rushing past us as we walk, more of the backdrop for our daily walks than what they really are, the ultimate destination which we seek?

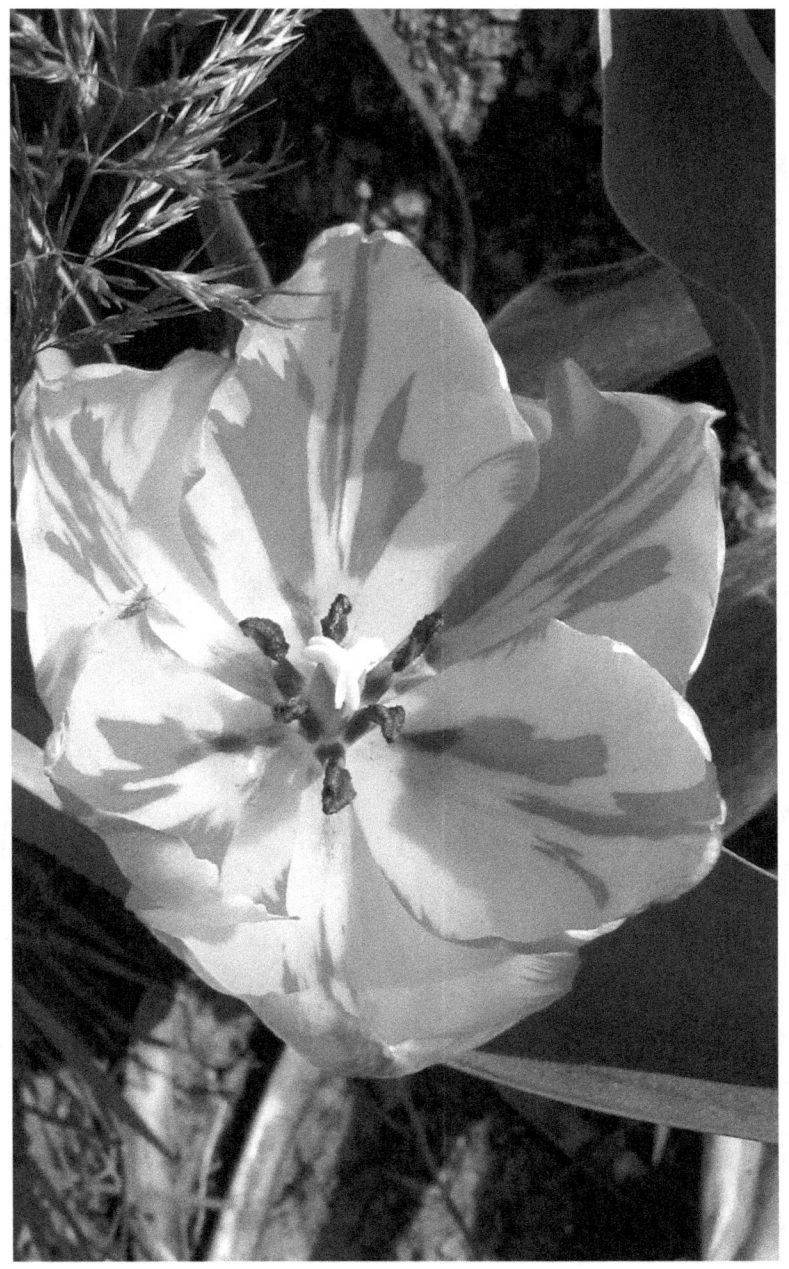

CHAPTER 20

WALKING WITH
A HIGHER PURPOSE

For many people who have a walking routine which addresses the needs of both mind and body, walking becomes something more than bodily exercise and an opportunity to rest the brain. While exercising the body and relaxing the mind is wonderful in its own right, there is often a natural progression to something more. After a time, the skills we learn through concentrated and mindful focus and the very act of taking these consistent mini-journeys out into the world as we cultivate our own secret garden of health and affirmation, begin to change the way we view our lives.

As our self-esteem builds we feel stronger as a person. Through our mind exercises we become more present and learn to keep mind chatter and negative thinking at bay. By physically moving our bodies through the physical world we develop a kinship with our environment and through mindfulness experiences learn to appreciate at a much deeper level the beauty and significance of our lives. Walking, something we once thought was a simple act insuring better health and longevity, becomes a powerful part of a personal myth which we reenact routinely and which then forms a connection with the long-existing human story of the individual hero's quest for change and transformation. Throughout time and in cultures in every corner of the globe we find a central story common to each human who walks upon this earth. That story while still alive in much of today's art and literature is not as vital to our culture as it once was in societies long ago or in the individual lives of the people who lived them. That story is the story of the hero, the man or woman who is motivated to get up and get moving, to set out on an initiatory journey which changes their lives and the lives of those around them.

In truth, each time we set out on our walks we are committing a revolutionary act, an act where the old order of status quo thought and behavior is slowly overturned. That which sits still grows stagnant, that which moves brings change; it's an old law, for activity stirs the pot and not only in the social order but within each of us as well. You may have noticed that this book is attempting to get you up and moving, and to encourage you to start participating in the creation of your own personal myth and the construction of a person who after their walk is different than the person they were before they started, someone who effects change not only in their own life but in the lives of those they touch. So what are the deep and fundamental principles underlying this central story, what is known among scholars as the great monomyth? Let's take a look.

From Ulysses to Jason, from Prometheus to Jesus and the Buddha, to even some of our cultural heroes of today, all share something in common: they fulfill the criteria of what it means to be a hero and therefore follow closely the general outline of the mythic hero or what has become known as world culture's monomyth, the age-old central story of the exceptional individual and their heroic life journey. Joseph Campbell wrote the seminal text on heroic myths, *Hero With a Thousand Faces*. In that book he defines a general pattern which is found in hero stories all over the world and throughout history. Campbell refers to that pattern in its simplest form as: Separation-----Initiation-----Return. The hero is living a status quo life at home then is suddenly moved by something to act; they then go through some form of initiation which deeply changes them and then return transformed to share what they have learned with those they have temporarily left behind.

It is possible to see something even as humble as our daily walk as a heroic journey, for like the heroes of old our journey initially starts with us living a routine lifestyle which unfortunately today is typically filled with stress, inactivity, and chaotic busyness, a lifestyle which makes it difficult for us to be healthy and to fully enjoy the gifts of life. Like many other heroes we learn that our lifestyle has become destructive to our mental and physical health and decide to separate ourselves from that injurious lifestyle long enough to seek out healing. Each walk itself becomes a form of initiation into a new lifestyle based in healthy exercise, mental focus and relaxation. The initiation is sometimes difficult but in the end transforming. When we return back to our homes we are changed, individuals with a new perspective, a perspective we value and want to share with those we know and love. As Campbell says, "… the successful adventure of the hero is the unlocking and release again of the flow of life into the body of the world."

Deep walkers walk the walk that all the heroes of history have walked before. To be personally changed, to bring a little new light into the world, one has to stop living their status quo lifestyle, get up, get out, and get moving. Yes, there are challenges to face, walking when we may not feel like it, inclement weather, a few aches and pains. But if the hero sticks with it there are immense benefits to be had, and there is no greater joy than sharing those benefits with others once our journey has begun and we notice change arising from somewhere deep within. There is no way to <u>transform</u> our lives without identifying with the central myth of the hero, for only through our deep walking initiation can we change the way we <u>see</u> our lives. As Campbell says in *Hero With a Thousand Faces,* "The objective world remains what it was, but, because of a shift of emphasis within, the subject is beheld as though transformed."

Once we have walked the hero's walk and completed what Campbell calls, "...a separation from the world, a penetration to some source of power, and a life-enhancing return," can we live life anew, healthier in both body and mind. So what is the mysterious "source of power" Campbell refers to in the quote above? In walking it is a wisdom we all possess and have unlimited access to, it is the wisdom of the natural body and insights of the natural mind. By distancing ourselves from the health-negating effects of our current lifestyles and focusing on life-affirming thoughts and actions, we have opened the doorway to a new life, a life we are now in control of and which renews our personal power.

While walking and working on our mind health using meditation techniques, it is possible to integrate our understanding of being on a personal heroic walk into our meditations as we take our walks, both those we take routinely and the one which lasts a lifetime. Nowhere have I found that integration better described than in a book by Thich Nhat Hanh, the Buddhist monk and Nobel Peace Prize nominee. In his book, *The Long Road Turns to Joy: A*

Guide to Walking Meditation, Hanh emphasizes the simplicity of walking meditation, something he says is available to everyone, for walking meditation is simply meditating while walking. It is something anyone can do, and something we should do with a smile and with a relaxed state of mind. Doing this, Hanh says, will make us feel "solid" as we walk the Earth, and our troubles will fall away as our hearts fill with joy. He says all it takes to gain the benefits of walking meditation is a little time and mindfulness, and the desire to be happy.

We must remember a very important principle as we practice walking meditation, and it is central to all forms of meditation. It is the principle of "seek <u>not</u> and ye shall find." People often assume that the goal of meditation is to find something which will give them inner peace, satori, or enlightenment. Nothing could be further from the truth. It is not about seeking something at all but more about allowing ourselves to recognize something we already have, something which completely surrounds us but which we fail to see. On this level, meditative walking is about walking, nothing more. It is we who complicate this simple act by projecting erroneous thoughts upon it, and make it far more complicated than it is. By describing it as a type of searching or seeking, we define it as something always out of reach. The truth is it has nothing to do with achievement or accomplishment, with getting something we do not already have, but with being. It has more to do with the discovery of our true nature, the very definition of satori, than searching and finding something beyond ourselves. The truth is that we are already enlightened. We have just covered our natural wisdom up with layers of non-being, with mental fast food and monkey chatter, with continual busyness and deleterious thinking.

When we walk, walk, nothing more. Be in the walking not in the thinking about walking. As the Buddha said, "When we walk, we know we are walking." And as A. J. Muste said, "There is no way to peace, peace is the way." In other words, there is no destination when we walk, walking is the destination.

Thich Nhat Hanh emphasizes in his book that as we walk we should walk with a smile on our face. This is the same smile which it is said the Buddha had as he walked and comes from the same understanding. It is a reflection of the deep and complete realization that we are alive and walking, and the understanding of what a true gift and privilege that is. We are not walking in our lives, "each step is life." If we begin to understand that each step is life, not the steps we have already taken or the steps we will take in the future, we will begin to live. Living happens now, in every instant of our conscious being. With each step we take, we arrive in the moment and Hanh says each time we truly arrive in the moment we become more secure and solid, and the more solid we are the greater sovereignty we have, which results in our being more free.

"Walking meditation is like eating." says Hanh. "With each step, we nourish our body and our spirit. When we walk with anxiety and sorrow, it is a kind of junk food. The food of walking meditations should be of a higher quality. Just walk slowly and enjoy the banquet of peace. "

Like many others, Hanh emphasizes the importance of gratitude, gratitude that we are blessed with being able to walk at all, and gratitude to be walking upon the earth at this time. This has become a primary focus in my own deep walking. When we walk mindfully in the moment a natural joyfulness begins to grow within, and also a realization of just how special it is to be able to be one of those capable of doing so. It becomes almost overwhelming and after a time it becomes impossible not to smile. When we come into the very center of our lives in the miracle of each present moment, we shed the peripheral spirit-numbing activities which for many of us constitute much of the substance of our daily lives. When we get away from a life defined by the stereotypical thinking which is generated by cultural clichés and simplistic thinking, it is like drinking from a clear cool stream, a stream which not only stems our thirst but sustains us. Have you ever taken a long hot hike in the mountains then stopped to drink from a mountain stream? It is in moments like these we feel most alive.

In the same way, when I am walking alone in a natural setting, totally focused on the present moment where I am a person alive and walking on this precious earth, I feel most vibrant and joyful. It is a total contrast to my return to the house where I unlace my shoes and sit down to watch the evening news, or look out my front window and see cars zipping in and out of the drive-thru fast-food restaurant down the street. We must never forget the privilege which the very act of walking is for as Hanh points out, "We walk for ourselves, and we walk for those who cannot walk. We walk for all living beings---past, present, and future."

When we take our "deep" walk, the way we walk is different than the way we walk during our daily routine. At least at first. Deep walking is not at all like sauntering to the store to pick up a few groceries or to slip outside to check the mail. It exists instead outside our daily routine and lives in a special dimension reserved for what we deeply value and respect. It is not some mindless stepping from point A to B but a sacred walk with special value, an act which symbolizes our self respect and appreciation for the gift we recognize our lives to be. Imagine for a moment that we were in immediate peril and at jeopardy to lose our lives. At that moment wouldn't we give anything to have one more opportunity to walk upon the Earth? At a time like that the simple act of walking would be seen for what it is: a privilege and a blessing.

Of course the truth is that we are all in immediate peril of losing our lives. Regardless of our age or fitness each of us could leave this mortal coil in an instant. All things come and go. And we remember that each time we put on our shoes and make the effort to get out and move. We move because we can. We walk because we believe that those who can walk should walk, that walking is the sign that we are not just alive but that we are active, active in our lives and actively demonstrating our respect for ourselves and our respect for life itself. If we begin to see our walking this way, it won't be long before even the walking which we do as part of our everyday lives will also be transformed into something mean- ingful and beautiful. For as Thich Nhat Hanh suggests, "Visualize a lotus, a tulip, a gardenia blooming under each step the moment your foot touches the ground. If you practice beautifully like this, your friends will see fields of flowers everywhere you walk."

We may well start taking routine walks for the health of our physical body, to lose weight, to strengthen our hearts, to live long enough to watch our grandchildren grow up. Yet soon our walks become important to us because not only do they make us feel more energetic, alive, and work as an antidote for potential illness, disease, and old age, but because they relax us, give us inner peace and serve as a kind of mental respite and counter balance to the mental stress we experience most of our day. Still, our walks are much more than this too, because the more one walks the more one's walk becomes. If we become a consistent walker it is almost impossible not to begin to realize that the simple daily walk we take not only makes us healthier and gives us peace of mind but becomes a metaphor for the "life walk" we all share, a kind of template for how to live each day, and an example of the deep connection we share with everything we encounter.

Over time, all the benefits we gain through walking will begin to influence our daily lives. Not only will we smile more, and value with deep mindfulness each person in our life, we will become more appreciative of the whole of life itself and see it for the miraculous endowment which it is. There are many paths to discover when we integrate walking into our lives, the path our feet follow as we head out the door, the path of our own new walking routine, the path to greater physical and mental health, the path which leads to self-discovery, the path of our lives as a whole. Remember, it takes many footsteps to form a path. The more steps we take to heal our bodies, the more steps we take to heal our minds, the easier it becomes to find our way on our own unique path and stay on that path over time. As Henry David Thoreau said long ago,

"As a single footstep will not make a path on the earth, so a single thought will not make a pathway in the mind. To make a deep physical path, we walk again and again. To make a deep mental path, we must think over and over the kind of thoughts we wish to dominate our lives."

CHAPTER 21

WALKING
THE WHOLE PERSON

As you may have noticed, while I have given you a variety of options for recommended mind activities while you are exercising your body, I have refrained from giving you detailed prescriptive walking instructions for each of your beginning or subsequent walks. Once you have learned the fundamentals, rather than having you follow my walks for you, I would rather have you use the many options I have given you and form them in a way that fits your abilities and needs. I do insist that we all do two things for the duration of our walks, leave negative thoughts behind and make a time and space for our special walking ritual which is our time of peace and healing. After that I encourage you to do the exercises in the order I have given them, at least initially, but beyond that, I hope you will get creative and discover what works best for you. Try a variety of the things I have suggested to see which are most effective. Do not try all of the mental exercises at once, certainly not on the same walk, or even in the same week or month. Do one at a time and master that one before moving on to the next. In truth, these exercises are the work of a lifetime and always a work in progress. Do give them time to work, and don't be afraid to mix them up to give your walks variety once you have worked on each of them individually. If you stick with your walking plan you will see it evolve over time into something deeply meaningful and fulfilling. When you make significant progress with your concentrated and mindful meditation techniques, work to increase the time you are able to spend in those states. But do give heed to the following warning.

Beware. Regular walking cannot only save your life, it can alter your life, so prepare for your life to be altered. Body movement is such a necessary biological need for us to remain healthy that if we do not move we not only jeopardize our lives but jeopardize the quality of our lives. Sure, without regular exercise you may still be breathing, but the truth of the matter is that breathing alone is not living.

Many people after integrating a walking program into their lives find many things begin to change. For instance, it is harder to continue to hold onto bad lifestyle habits. In fact, there is an interesting dynamic between positive and negative lifestyle habits: they have a hard time coexisting. They are the opposite of each other, and often times opposites do not attract. True, one occasionally sees them trying to exist together. In fact, the other day I saw a man actually smoking a cigarette as he laced up his jogging shoes and prepared to go for a run. Still, I think we all know that at some point in that man's life either the cigarettes or jogging shoes will have to go.

Getting regular exercise is a true life or death decision and once you opt for life many life-negating behaviors other than your past inactive lifestyle will begin disappearing and be replaced by behaviors which are more life-affirming. Again as Dr. Stewart suggests everything in our lives is either health-denying or health-affirming, and while they can exist side by side, more often then not they tend to settle out and become mostly one or the other, promoting better health or promoting illness. Remember, even one bad health habit tends to open the door for other unhealthy habits just as healthy habits tend to inspire more healthy habits.

Dr. Stewart lists eight items in *Deep Medicine* which he believes are necessary for a healthy life for both body and mind, and do not be surprised if after walking consistently for a time you begin to crave and seek out some of the other things on Dr. Stewart's list.

1. A balanced diet
2. Regular exercise
3. Time for play, fun, and laughter
4. Music, singing, chanting, and dancing
5. Love, touch, relationships, and support networks
6. Engaging in creative pursuits in work and leisure
7. Time spent in nature, with beauty, and in healing environments
8. Faith and belief in the sacred, spiritual, or unknowable

Why would many of these other things become attractive to us once we begin to get our health back? It's because all of these things are the hallmarks of a healthy life, a life which a healthy body and mind require to function optimally. Once we begin to participate in one healthy activity it can have a snowballing effect. Few people will go out for a half hour walk through a beautiful setting in the fresh air, come home exhilarated and full of life then sit down to a snack of milk and cookies or pour themselves a large martini. In the way that downward spirals maintain their energy or even intensify their energy in an ever-increasing downward spiral movement by cannibalistically feeding on themselves, upward spirals tend to do something similar but in a different way, spiraling upward ever faster by building upon themselves. Don't be surprised if after going on a good mind/body walk you get home and feel like a simple glass of cool clear water with a piece of raw vegetable or fruit; change is a beautiful thing.

The goal of eventually walking the whole person means that we recognize that we as individuals are greater than the sum of our parts, that we are healthier when all of our parts are on the same page, working together in a beautiful unity of body, heart, mind, and spirit. A consistent walking regimen is often the first step, a critically important step, which can give our lives momentum in a profoundly new and positive direction. As I said in the introduction, I hope this book will help you take that first step, and I encourage you to do so. But you alone will have to take it, putting one foot in front of the other and moving forward step by step, walk by walk. Again, a body at rest often wants to stay at rest, but on the positive side, a body in motion has a tendency to want to stay in motion. In fact this book was designed not only to be a probe, prodding you to get up and take that first step, it was designed to follow the stages of your walk as well, a walk that starts primarily as a body health activity then progresses into the realm of emotional, mental, and even moral and spiritual health. It follows the pattern of the development I wish for you, a life walk culminating in the creation of a more integrated person, one who is happier and healthier and whose majority of habits and activities are life affirming rather than life negating. So let's take a moment and lace-up our walking shoes and take an imaginary walk together.

As we tie up our laces (I double knot mine) let's think first about how far we have come just by starting this walk together. We have learned about the growing epidemic of inactivity for which "Walking is man's best medicine," and learned that a body at rest tends to stay at rest and risks the possibility of advancing to permanent rest, resting in peace. The very fact that we are tying up our shoes indicates that we have chosen not to let inactivity diminish the quality or duration of our lives. The list of diseases we become susceptible to by being inactive continually echoes in our minds and pushes us out the front door becoming our first mantra. So lets chant it aloud together,

"Anxiety, cardiovascular disease, depression, cancer, high blood pressure, obesity, osteoporosis, lipid disorders, kidney stones."

An odd mantra I know, but a mantra none-the-less, the only negative mantra we are allowed to use, one that motivates us by reminding us of the things we want to avoid. But from here on out only positive thoughts are allowed. As we step outside into the natural world we say aloud our second walking mantra: "I choose to move...I choose to move." All the excuses we once recited to exempt us from doing something for our health have faded away. "I don't have time," is gone. "I can't afford it," is gone. "I have more important things to do," gone. We have seen through our own impotent attempts to excuse ourselves from the one thing we should be doing for ourselves and for those whose lives are interwoven with our own. We are doing what is right and responsible, we are choosing to make our bodies move. After having already worn a pedometer for a few weeks, reality is now staring us in the face and forces us to swallow a bitter truth: "We have fallen into a lifestyle which is becoming more and more sedentary, and our low activity level has become a life habit which is literally costing us our lives." But there is only one conclusion we can come to now, proven by the action of lacing up our shoes, we now choose life over premature death and choose to make our bodies homes where greater health resides rather than being homes of sickness, anxiety and despair.

It feels good to stretch. We know that we have to start our walking habit gradually, that our bodies are not used to this yet and at first we must be sure to keep it a fun and positive experience, careful not to do too much too soon. As we do our knee curls and side reaches we think about what this stretching does, mostly warming up our muscles and increasing our flexibility. But we recognize too that in a sense we are stretching our inner selves as well, encouraging our bodies and minds to do more than they are accustomed to doing, coaxing them to walk resolutely toward the realm of better health. We are literally stretching ourselves in every way, and by so doing not only increasing our strength and flexibility but realizing the whole of our human potential. It feels good to stretch. Yes, of course there is a just a little discomfort, for there is some discomfort in all growth as we move out of the sameness of habitual routine and comfort and become something more, something much more. When we realize this, any little ache and pain we feel is seen as a sign that we are choosing to increase the boundaries of our being, an act of stretching which will end in increased happiness and health, and the smile we feel growing on our face is a reflection of a new joy as it begins to grow within.

We have agreed not to talk on our walk together today. We want to focus on something more important, on the feelings and thoughts which arise as we walk without the influence of the words and thoughts of others. As we think about the issue of walking alone like a warrior or walking together as members of common tribe we realize that we can do both simultaneously, by walking alone together.

We stand still for a second after warming up then take our first step forward. And what a step it is. It is the first step in what will be according to our pedometers the first of 4000 steps in our walk this morning, but which is also the first step in what will be a succession of hundreds of thousands of steps over the years ahead as we continue to walk our walk. Again as they say, a journey of a thousand miles begins with a single step, well, the journey to health, happiness, and joy begins with a single step as well, and that first step is one of the most important of our lives because it will determine the quality of the life we enjoy in what life we have left to live. It's one small step in the moment, one giant leap for the rest of our lives.

As we take our first steps on what Thich Nhat Hanh calls "the long road (which) turns to joy" we leave our daily world behind. We move not so much away from our homes of comfort and stability in order to escape them, but in order to move toward something new and transforming which in the end we will return with to our homes to the benefit of all those we know. In so doing we focus mostly not on what we are moving away from but on what we are moving towards, a new and dramatically revitalized life forever altered. We keep one eye on the present and one eye on where it will lead us but only a suspect eye on the past which has in part defined us and now can also limit us. It is new ground we are breaking and the old ground which would if we allowed it try to pull us back into the stagnant world we have left behind, is itself left behind. For the moment we will stay in the moment and forget not only the distant past but the immediate past with its tiring and endless rush, pressure and push, endless deadlines, constant demands, and focus mindfully on the simple yet elegant movement of our bodies in space as we engage in the simple act of human walking. Any negative thoughts or even any thoughts about anything that existed before this current moment are allowed to simply evaporate from our consciousness as we focus instead on the miracle we experience, our bodies in movement, the sound of our breathing, the footsteps moving us ahead. "This is my body moving...this is my body moving..." is the mantra which now comes naturally to mind. "Each step renews me...each step renews me..." the affirmation which now springs spontaneously to our lips. "Each step I take leads me closer to my self."

As we move further down the trail we are careful not to focus on goals, knowing that what we achieve is achieved in the here and now and not at some distant date and time. The miracle is now, the reward is in the moment, better health the result of our moving our bodies consistently in time and of totally surrendering to the beauty of that. Our goal is no goal, for we need nothing more than this. What we have if we appreciate it fully and use it correctly is enough. If we have any goal at all it is to enjoy each step of our walk; where it takes us is of secondary concern. If we walk with the proper attitude wherever our walk ends will be the right place for it to end. We need to keep it light, keep it easy, and keep it fun. We never walk with a scowl or grimace on our face, but replace it with the Buddha's all-knowing smile.

Do you feel that too? The way the world begins to change? With every step we take our Secret Garden grows around us and negative thoughts slip away, returning to the now distant realm we have left behind. This is our space which we alone create, our sacred ground for growth and change. Our primary intent is to appreciate it as it is and to stand back and watch it all unfold. Now we mindfully watch each leg lift up and step forward; we watch each thought arise and fade, for we are both the gardener and the guard, planting seeds of positive thought, not allowing any toxic weeds to grow, sensing the body's response to movement and being mindful as our bodies move. Do you feel your silent witness forming, the one who stands above it all, who simply watches everything unfold while focusing on the positive and filtering out the negative in a light-handed and compassionate way? While we want all voices to speak to us, from the complaints and joys of bodily sensation to the complaints and joys of mind, we emphasize and encourage only the constructive ones to stay, for as we walk through our Secret Garden we never forget our true destination, increased renewal, permanent healing, and joy.

Look over there! They call that thing a tree, that stuff beneath our feet, the earth. But how can each of these miraculous things be reduced to single words like these? Earth, and tree? For a moment let's try to walk without attaching mind symbols to the world we see. As we walk let's not think "sky, lake, tree, flower, and earth;" we see much more than this and realize that words really can't describe the miracle we are walking through.

We choose the words we allow in our minds carefully. Monkey chatter is left behind and replaced with simple affirmations, then words are allowed only to describe the details of our bodies as they move: "Lift leg, step forward, touch the ground."

Now let's take a moment to move out of our brains and bodies and into the world around us. Let's try to transition out of the world of thought, even mindful thought, and into the world of basic being. How do we feel about the environment around us? What things are our senses attracted to? Is it the feel of the earth beneath our feet or any trees or flowers we see along the path? We try to see each object from the viewpoint of a child or someone come from another world who is overwhelmed by what their eyes reveal of the new world in their view. How does the world look from this perspective? Let's try to make the world we take for granted regain its novel magnificence and see if we can regain our original sense of awe and wonder. We think of Thoreau and his love of the country in contrast to the town, and his belief that everything in the natural world promotes our health, every delicate gust of wind blowing through every leaf of tree.

Lets now return for a moment to word thought with a few more affirmations, letting them come in a rhythm which matches our footsteps. We will let these words into our consciousness not so much to describe the world for us, but to fill us up with positive thoughts about the experience we are having. "When I walk I am free...when I walk I am free..." Make up your own affirmation now and let the words which you are saying work their way deep inside of you. "When I walk I am alive...when I walk I choose to live..." As we walk now let's try to slip between the two different mind states, first experiencing the world with few or ideally no words parading through our heads, then, when we start to let the words back in, make sure they are only those which richly avow the beauty of the new world we create.

We are feeling a bit exceptional now you and I, somewhat like heroes as we walk together through this beautiful day, sharing our footpath with those heroes who walked before. Our simple little walk is like all great walks throughout all time and we stand on the shoulders of great women and men who have taken the walk before us. Something has moved us to act, to get up off the couch and out of the house and that something is the search for health in body and mind, the true treasure we seek on our personal mythic quest. We recognize that each walk is a mini-search for that, and all of our walks add-up together to form a longer walk which seeks the same. Soon that longer walk becomes itself the foundation of our lives where each walk we take becomes not a journey to some distant destination but is itself the destination which we seek. Like all the heroes before us we learn that our journey really lies within and the challenges we face are nothing but the mythic monsters we create.

Can you feel at depth as I do that better health is our natural state? A place where the body and mind prefer to be, where they are most comfortable and where they operate optimally in a form of human homeostasis? Much like water we seek our own natural level with the body seeking improved health and the mind seeking greater peace. And we feel at last our minds and bodies working together, there is no mind/body split, our bodies listen to an affirming mind, and our minds let our bodies reintroduce us to the wisdom of our bones and flesh. We have learned too that most often we are the ones who have made the choices which have blocked our way, stood between us and the healthy life we seek. So as we move forward step by step on today's walk, and continue stepping forward in every walk we take, we too exterminate dragons along the way which threaten us from all corners, dragons of our own creation, created by lifestyle choices and our own lack of knowledge and wisdom. At last we learn what all heroes learn: that which we seek has been here all along, and our inability to see it is not because we have not looked hard enough but because we have been too blind to see what has been right in front of us all along. As true heroes we must at last admit, when we met the enemy he was us.

Once this new understanding enters our lives we begin to understand that the little walk we share today is a paradigm for the big walk, the very walk of life itself; we begin to take what we learn in the little walk and apply those truths to the larger one. We generally stop pointing fingers at others and accept full responsibly for the quality of our daily walk and current life walk as well, pointing the finger of blame or credit where we should, directly at the center of our chests. Once we take responsibility for our health and we define health as all we think, feel, and do, what then is left to blame on others? We are the heroes in our own central myth; there is no one to live our lives but us; it is our choice in the end, for who will be our hero if not ourselves?

Inside of us now a new feeling grows. It is the recognition that it is an honor to walk this walk, both the walk from cradle to grave and each daily walk we take. It is a privilege. We should never think of it as a small thing; there really is nothing greater. For when we walk we walk not only for ourselves but for everyone who has ever walked before or ever will walk when we are gone. We walk for those alive today who cannot walk due to ill health or injury. For them it is inconceivable that someone like you and I who are capable of walking would ever choose not to do so, for walking is the ultimate celebration of life itself. When we try to determine if something is alive or dead we wait to see if it will move. Life without movement is no life at all; so for all who can't walk, for all who once walked but walk no more, for those who will one day walk where we now walk, we walk for them. And I hope that when we are gone others will come along to walk for us. We are part of a continuous river of walkers walking into life then walking back into the common ocean from which we've come. Just like a thought we come and go, suddenly born into being only to fade away, still we don't fear death. We are a part of a greater cycle now, and as someone once said, it is after all not death which we should fear, but fear instead having never lived our lives.

Not only is walking the ultimate expression of living, it puts us in contact with our ultimate being. Thich Nhat Hanh suggests that there are two primary dimensions to life, the waves and the water. He notes that the ocean's surface is made up of waves, some large and small, some beautiful and inspiring and others violent and threatening, some holding shape, others quickly disappearing, waves that build and fall as others rise up to replace them. But he says if we touch each wave deeply we realize that they are all made of the same thing: water, for all individual waves originate from the same sea. "From the point-of-view of the water," Hanh says, "there is no beginning, no end, no up, no down, no birth, and no death." Walking he believes, if we do it with mindfulness within the present moment, connects us to the water of life rather than to the waves of life, and that's why every place where our feet touch the earth a beautiful flower grows.

So walk on and walk deeply my friend; we will always walk this walk together. Be sure to make your own pathway in the world and don't follow the path of another. As Ralph Waldo Emerson said, "Do not go where the path may lead, go instead where there is no path and leave a trail." And remember too the Buddha's words, "You cannot truly travel the path until you have become the path itself."

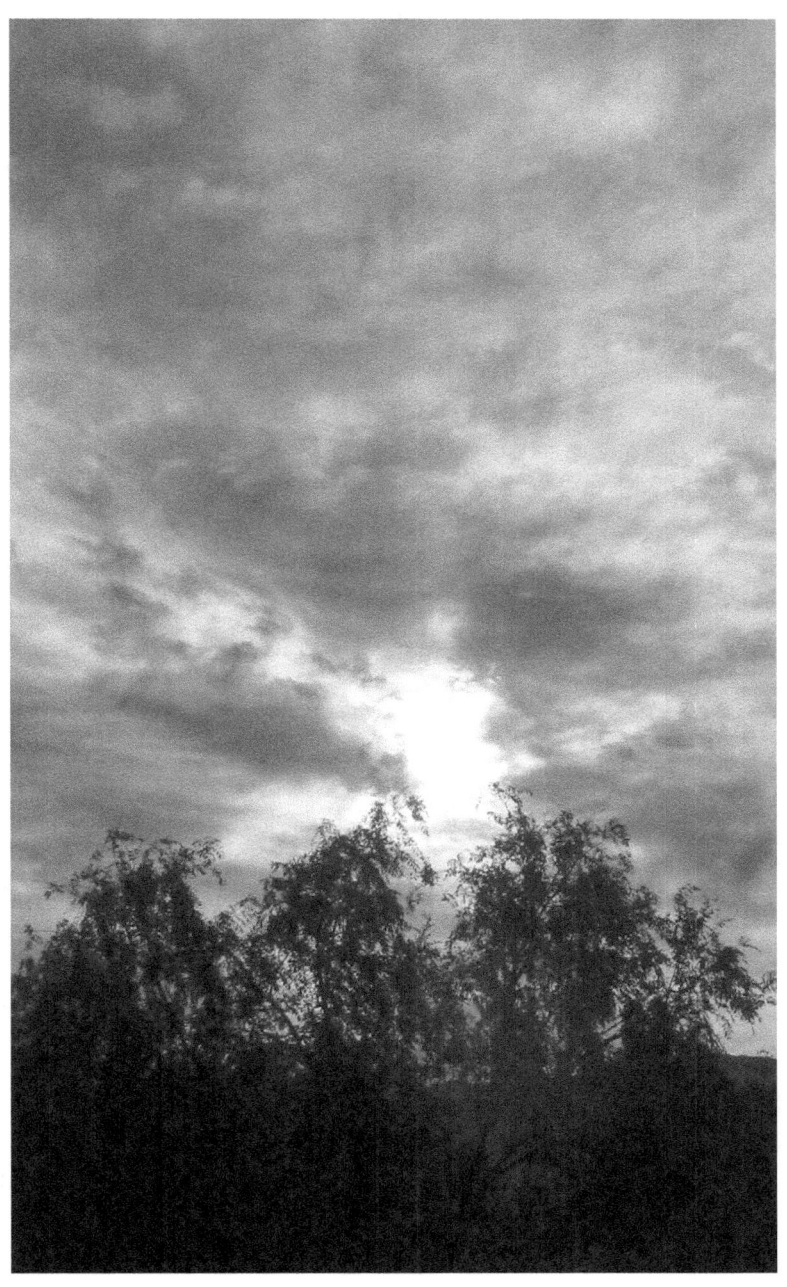

KEEPING RECORD

There are some important things for us to keep track of as we first begin then continue our walking regimen. These things are how often we walk, how long we walk, and the changes we feel in body and mind before, during, and after we walk. To track these things we need to set up a little walking journal which is part calendar and part diary. I recommend that we get a notebook to which we can add pages, perhaps a small three ring binder. Once we have one, we will divide it into three sections. The first section contains a calendar where we write down the number of steps or miles we travel each day based on our pedometer readings. The second section is used to make short dated entries on how our body responded to our walk, our physical feelings before, during and after our walk, and a third journal section where we record how our minds responded to that walk, our developing ability to keep negative thoughts away, and our response to any meditative activities we try. Let me discuss those three sections in a little more detail.

Our Calendar

Whether we choose to use a day planner or a calendar it does not have to be attached to our three ring notebook, but it should at least be kept inside of it or close by. In the beginning, each day we walk we will want to record the total number of steps we have taken for the whole day. For a time those numbers should include our step count for the days we do not take a walk so we can see the contrasting numbers. After a time, once we know we are averaging around 10,000 steps per day consistently we can free ourselves from our pedometers and simply write down the amount of time we walk each time we walk. Another option is that since a person takes about 2,000 steps for every mile they walk we can write down our totals in either steps, miles, or the amount of time walked. Before long we will learn when we need to supplement our daily activity with a walk, and how much of a walk we need, based on our understanding of approximately how many steps we take each day without going out for a walk. But in the beginning, our calendar and daily entries will help keep us honest and encourage us each time we look at our calendar and see the number or our daily entries begin to multiply.

After a year or even after a few months it can be exhilarating to leaf through our calendar and see it all marked up and realize that all of those markings represent our effort to transform our life. They are visual testimony to our commitment and to the strength of our conviction. Our calendar markings also makes it easy to see any blank areas and gives us an idea about how well we have done with our walking consistency. Like most people we will have some holes and some longer blank areas on our calendars occasionally. When we see them we need to cut ourselves some slack but then try to create a calendar the following month or year which gives us even more pride when we look at them. In other words, in the beginning, pay attention to the inconsistencies, accept that we are human, but work to have a calendar with more consistent entries in the future. We are all a work in progress and always will be. When friends stop by we can show them our marked up calendars and say, "Look, isn't it beautiful?" If they return our question with a puzzled look don't worry, at least you and I will understand the beauty which we see.

<u>Our Daily Diary</u>

The diary portion of our record keeping will have two basic sections: one titled *Walking Body* where we record how our bodies respond to both the last walk we have completed and to our developing walking program as a whole, and a section titled *Walking Mind* where we record our mind activities on our last walk and any changes to our general mindset we have noticed since we started keeping record. Our written entries need to both express generalizations about these things but also provide specific examples. Therefore an entry might include, "I felt invigorated, happy, and healthy," but then provide more detail, "I could feel the blood pumping to my heart and hear myself breathing, each breath made me feel more solid and free." We will want to present examples of our thoughts, including the challenges we overcome to keep them positive, the mental activities we worked on, and how we felt we did with those activities on our last walk and over the entire period of time we have been walking consistently. "At first I found it difficult to keep my mind on walking. I worried about the problems I was having with the kids, but soon after I began to walk I focused on the rhythm of my foot strikes and on the way the light was coming through the surrounding trees." We need to do our best to make our writing something that we will find interesting and fun to read if we choose to read it in the future. We will find that by reviewing our journals which record our struggles and successes it will help keep us motivated and demonstrate to us in our own writing and words the dramatic changes we are experiencing in both body and mind.

The length of our journal entries is up to each of us. Rather than making this a chore, we write in our journals only when we are genuinely motivated to do so. Writing in our journal is not meant to be so much a discipline as a joyous and creative out-pouring of our thoughts and feeling about the healthful activity we have chosen for ourselves. Trust me, soon you will begin to want to tell everyone you know about it; we just need to tell our journals first. Here are a few more details on what we want these journal sections to look like.

In both the body and mind sections we want to be sure to assign a date to our entry. We want to see a chronological progression and the evolution of our thoughts and feelings. In the body section as we relate how our bodies are responding to our walking program we will want to discuss as many elements of our physical experience as we can. I am not suggesting we do so for each and every walk or for even one walk, but do try to cover all aspects of a walk over time. In this way we will build for ourselves a comprehensive and detailed description of our walking experience from start to finish.

What does it feel like to be stretching before we begin? How is our flexibility at the moment and how are we feeling overall?

Are our bodies tired after we walk or invigorated and did we find the walk difficult or easy? Soon we will notice a change in how our bodies feel, and notice a slight difference in each individual walk and the powerful cumulative effect we experience with the more walks we complete. We can also detail how each part of our bodies respond, from legs to lungs, from arms to heart and all the body parts in between. Again we will want to be specific but also include a general assessment about our body's overall response to the increased amount of movement we have chosen for ourselves.

In the *Walking Mind* section of our journal over time we need to be sure to describe our mental state during our walk from start to finish as well. What are we thinking before we start our walk, as we lace-up our shoes? Are we excited about getting started or feeling dread? Is there any change in our mental state after our walk begins or does it remain constant? How are we doing with creating our "secret garden?" Are we able to keep negative thinking out of our heads? If so, how did we do it? If not, how do we plan to change that?

It is beneficial to record our mental experiences when we try affirmations or any of the other positive thought activities or meditation techniques. We should record our mental response to the way our body feels and interacts with the sensual world around it, and write about any changes in our mental state throughout the duration of our walk and try to identify what if anything contributed to that change. Again, we want to record the little shifts that occur mentally as we walk and also try to identify the overall effect of our walking has had on our mental state even during the times we are not walking. Are we starting to see any positive benefits our mental exercises are having at other times?

It is important that we be honest in all of our journal entries. These journal entries are for us and will help us see the way our minds and bodies are changing through regular exercise. While we want to keep a positive attitude about what we are doing, we don't want to fake it. It is as normal to have variation in our mental responses to walking as it is to have variation in our body's responses to those walks. These variations are normal. While we may aspire to be the water rather than the waves, understand that the waves we feel with their up and down swings are in part the natural ebb and flow of life and have a beauty all their own. While our inner witness may stand above carefully watching, it learns to accept and enjoy it all.

APPENDIX 2

IF YOU STOP AND CAN'T
GET RESTARTED

Don't worry, everyone stops from time to time. I like to think of it
as simply varying the time between our walks rather than viewing
it as permanently ending our walking routine. We should think of
it as resting longer between our walks rather than scaring ourselves
with thoughts of possibly ending our hard-earned walking regimen
forever. After all if we never stopped walking between our walks
we would be walking around all the time wouldn't we? Be it stopping due to illness, because of a walking injury, because company
has come to visit and is living in our home, or just because we have
slipped out of the walking habit for a while, at some point almost
everyone has times when they are walking more or less, and stopping for longer or shorter periods of time between their walks.

How we think of our stopping is what will determine if we
begin to walk again after a short hiatus or if we settle back into
a lifestyle which includes far more sitting and much less moving.
Since we are all very skilled excuse makers, we may even use
the fact that we have stopped as a way to excuse ourselves from

returning to a walking routine. We do this by making our stopping into a much bigger deal than it really is, and using it to show ourselves that a walking regimen was really not for us in the first place, that we tried it but it just didn't work. We focus on the fact of how hard we tried rather than focusing on how hard we didn't try and thereby don't have to focus on the problem of having stopped in the first place or figuring out how to get going again. By telling ourselves that we tried it and it wasn't for us, we put the blame on the walking activity itself and not on ourselves. After all, we tried didn't we? We did <u>our</u> part. It just wasn't our thing.

If we do stop walking on a consistent basis regardless of the reason, we may find it difficult to start our walking routine again. Even if we stop for just a week and have already experienced many of the benefits of a regular walking program, it is sometimes hard to get our momentum up again. But it does seem that we sometimes give our temporary stopping a kind of significance and power beyond its due, so we must always remember the powerful lure of sedentary inertia and the manipulative reasoning of our inner nay-sayer. Even a stoppage for a week or so can make our body at rest want to remain at rest and start the nay-sayer whispering in our ear once again all the reasons we should stay still.

At a time like this we close our ears to the excuse maker (we have succeeded in quieting him before) and remember that this stopping time can actually have positive benefits. Yes, it is a time when we are at risk for stopping our walking program completely and that should not be underestimated, but it is also a chance to reevaluate what our walking program has done for us and use our new understanding of how our own minds work to move forward. We already know well how our minds are capable of using both negative and positive thinking to either urge us back on track or encourage us off track once again. We have seen how the little health-negator on one of our shoulders has tried to tempt us before and now he may want to tempt us back into the great stillness once again. But we have an advantage this time. We have with our new perspective and inner witness watched our own thinking move between the poles of positive and negative, and the little internal discourager has nothing to say we haven't heard before. This is just a new version of the old self-generated con game we have fought against throughout our lives and now once again floods our brains with all the reasons we should stop consistent walking for good.

Fortunately this time we are wiser, for this time we see the bigger picture and are no longer blind to our own self-sabotaging behaviors. We accept that we stop after an individual walk and we accept that sometimes we stop walking for a longer period of time between them. That does not mean that we abandon the larger picture, the picture of us on our walking path, a path meandering throughout our life regardless of how often we stop, when we stop, and for however long we stop. In a way, stopping will always be a part of walking, just as stillness is forever a part of movement, and silence a necessary ingredient of sound. And we can use that still- ness and silence to create an even more beautiful music in which to walk than we have ever enjoyed before. We don't fear stillness, we don't fear silence, and we don't fear stopping. Wouldn't it be silly to suddenly stand still and assume we might never move again or hear a musical rest in a beautiful song and conclude that it had ended?

So, when we stop due to a change of schedule like an impromptu vacation, a new family routine, a change of job, or illness or for some other reason, think of that stopping as the pause between one beautiful note and a beautiful note yet to be played, and understand that that silence is an integral part of every song. It is also an opportunity to reassess why we started walking consistently in the first place, and the benefits it has already given us. This occasional assessment is something we should do even if we don't stop walking for a period of time longer than usual.

In fact the time we take to pause in our walking routine is the perfect time to reread our Walking Diary, an opportunity to remind ourselves of what we have accomplished and the benefits we have gained. It will help us to once more appreciate what walking has already done for us and remind us of the gifts it has for us in the future. Stopping should make us appreciate it more and have us looking forward to getting back to regular walking once again. While we are stopped let's remember with the help of our diary the challenges we have already overcome and the joys and benefits we have reaped, and rather than shaming our selves like we may have in the past, just quiet our minds and lace-up our shoes.

Because we have already come to understand that each daily walk is really just a part of our life-long walk, and that our walking regimen is a metaphor for the walk of life itself, we realize what stopping our daily walking means. We wouldn't give-up and stop walking the walk of life would we? All of our walks and succession of walks are always about the big things and small, about starting and stopping, about walking's pleasures and temptations, its challenging times and comforting times and moments of overwhelming joy. What we learn about dealing with all those things will help sustain us, and sustain our walking program as well.

Once we do successfully overcome a stopping episode, it will make it easier to overcome any that follow. We will see future stops differently. Once, through mental focus and a new understanding we overcome the whole issue of stop and non-stop, stepping forward or standing still, we will have had a personal victory which will benefit us in analogous events in other aspects of our lives. Be it eating poorly when we are trying to eat right, giving up on a project instead of seeing it through, dropping out of an important relationship instead working on it, once we have successfully defeated the defeatist dynamic even in something as simple as daily walking we will be able to see it more clearly in the future and conquer it more easily in all aspects of our lives.

The secret to conquering a defeatist attitude in all circumstances is ultimately the same, and that is not to succumb to life's daily ebb and flow, but always keep the bigger picture in sight. Remember, we are not the waves we are the water, and we are not the sum total of our individual walks or the time we rest between them. We are now for the rest of our lives, Life Walkers, despite the length of our walks or the duration of our stops. So get out and try a new walking path for variety, or just walk every other day for a week or two, or buy yourself some new walking shoes. Whatever it takes to help you head out the door is precisely what you need to do. I have no doubt that I will see you again on the walking path we both cherish, and if you love life as I do and carefully listen on your next walk, you may hear me singing words of encouragement to you to remind you of the reason we came here in the first place, "staying alive, staying alive..."

RESOURCE MATERIAL

Barbor, Cary. 2001. "The Science of Meditation." Article. <u>Psychology Today</u>.

Blair, Steven N. 2009. "Physical Inactivity: The Biggest Public Health Problem of the 21st Century." British Journal of Sports Medicine. Vol. 43, Issue 1.

Bonadonna R. 2003. "Meditation's impact on chronic illness." *Holistic Nursing Practice* ;17(6):309–319.

Boone, J. E., Gordon-Larsen, Penny, Adair, Linda S., Popkin, Barry M. 2007. "Screen time and physical activity during adolescence: longitudinal effects on obesity in young adulthood." <u>International Journal of Behavioral Nutrition and Physical Activity</u>.

Bumgardner, Wendy. 2012. "Walking for your mind and spirit." Article. [Online] About.com. http://walking.about.com/cs/mindandspirit/a/mindspirit.htm.

Campbell, Joseph. 2008. *The Hero With a Thousand Faces*. Novato, Ca. New World Library. Third Ed. Print.

Campbell, Joseph. 2004. *Pathways to Bliss*. New World Library. Print.

Carr, Nicholas. 2011. *The Shallows: What the Internet is Doing to Our Brains*. New York. W.W. Norton & Co. Print.

Cissell, Michelle A., Ph.D. 2012. "Don't Sweat It! Exercise and Type 1 Diabetes." Article. Juvenile Diabetes Research Foundation.

Cohen, Sheldon; Janicki-Deverts, D; Miller, Gregory, E.; 2007. "Psychological Stress and Disease." Journal of the American Medical Association.

Crowley, Chris. & Henry S. Lodge, M.D. *Younger Next Year*. New York. Workman Publishing. 2004. Print.

Davidson, R.J.; Kabat-Zinn, J.; Schumacher, J.; et al. 2003. "Alterations in brain and immune function produced by mindfulness meditation." *Psychosomatic Medicine*; 65(4):564–570.

Dietz, William H. 1996. "The Role of Lifestyle in Health: The Epidemiology and Consequences of Inactivity." Proceedings of the Nutrition Society. Oxford University Press.

Dorn, Joan. 2012. "Getting Fit: Why More People Are Walking The Walk." NPR Transcript.

"EMedtv." 2012. Benefits of Walking." Article [Online] http://weight-loss.emedtv.com/exercise/benefits-of-walking.html

Fredrik, P. 2012. "100 benefits of meditation." I Need Motivation: Excellence in Life Enrichment. [Online] http://www.ineedmotivation.com/blog/2008/05/100-benefits-of-meditation/

Fremantle, Francesca. 2003. *Luminous Emptiness*. Boston & London. Shambhala Press.

Galper, Daniel I. ; et al. 2006. "Inverse Association between Physical Inactivity and Mental Health in Men and Women." *Medicine & Science in Sports & Exercise*. Vol. 38 - Issue 1.

Hanh, Thich Nhat. 1996. *The Long Road Turns To Joy*. Berkeley, Ca., Parallax Press. Print.

Hawking, Steven. 2010. *The Grand Design*. New York, New York. Bantam Books. Print.

Hu, Frank B.; Li, Tricia Y.; Colditz, Graham A. 2003. "Television watching and other sedentary behaviors in relation to risk of obesity and Type 2 diabetes mellitus in women." *Journal of the American Medical Association*.

Keleman, Stanley. 1981. *Your Body Speaks Its Mind*. Berkeley, Ca. Center Press. Print.

King, Alexandra. 2012. "Health risks of physical inactivity similar to smoking." *Nature Reviews Cardiology* 9.

Kravitz, Len. Ph.D. 2007. "The 25 Most Significant Health benefits of Physical Activity & Exercise." *IDEA Health & Fitness Association*. Article.

Landers, Dr. Daniel. 2006. "The Influence of Exercise on Mental Health." *Research Digest*.

Lutz, A.; Slagter, H. A.; Dunne, J.; et al. 2008. "Attention regulation and monitoring in meditation." *Trends in Cognitive Sciences*.:12(4);163–169.

Mann; Hosman; Schaalma; and de Vries. 2004. "Self-esteem in a broad-spectrum approach for mental health promotion." *Oxford Journals*. Vol. 19. Issue 4.

Marano, Hara Estroff. 2001. "Move to boost mood." *Psychology Today*.

Mayo Clinic Staff. 2011. "Walking: Trim your waistline, improve your health." Article [Online] http://www.mayoclinic.com/health/walking/HQ016

Meditation and Health. [Report] Centers for disease Control and Prevention. [Online] http://www.cdc.gov/features/meditation/

Miller, Lyle H.; Smith, Alma Dell. 2012. *The Stress Solution*. Review in American Psychological Association Magazine.

"Nature Therapy-Walking in Nature." 2012. Article. [Online] Squidoo.com. http://www.squidoo.com/nature-therapy.

Navratilova, Martina. 2010. "Walking: The Easiest Exercise." From AARP.

Newland, Guy. 2008. *Introduction to Emptiness*. Ithaca, N.Y. Snow Lion Publications. Print.

"Obesity Related Statistics in America." 2012. Get America Fit Foundation. Article. [Online] http://www.getamericafit. org/statistics-obesity-in-america.html.

Otto, Michael Ph.D. ; Smits, Jasper Ph.D. 2011. 'Exercise for Mood and Anxiety.' Oxford University Press, Inc. Fotheringham, Michael J. ; Wonnacott, Rebecca L. ; Owen, Nevile. 2000. "Computer Use and Physical Inactivity in Young Adults: Public Health Perils and Potentials of New Information Technologies. *Annals of Behavioral Medicine*. Vol. 22-Issue 4.

Paluska, S. A. ; Schwenk, T. L. 2000. "Physical Activity and Mental Health: Current Concepts." *Sports Medicine*. Vol. 29, Number 3.

Penedo, Frank J; Dahn, Jason R. 2005. "Exercise and Well-being: A Review of Mental and Physical Health Benefits Associated with Physical Activity". *Current Opinion in Psychiatry*. Vol. 18-Issue 2.

"Physical Inactivity: A Global Health Problem." World Health Organization. [Online] http://www.who.int/dietphysicalactivity/factsheet_in activity/en/

Powell, K. E. ; Blair, S. N. 2012. "The public health burdens of sedentary living habits; theoretical but realistic estimates." Europe PubMed Central.

"Prevalence of Sedentary Leisure-time Behavior Among Adults in the United States." 1997. Article. [Online] Centers for Disease Control and Prevention. http://www.cdc.gov/nchs/data/hestat/sedentary/sedentary.htm

Price, Cynthia J., Ph.D.; Thompson, Elaine A., Ph.D., Measuring Dimensions of Body Connection: Body Awareness and Body Dissociation. 2011. PMC, U.S. National Library of Medicine National Institutes of Health.

Puff, Robert Ph.D. "Reflections on Meditation: A guide for Beginners." E-book. [Online] http://www.eBookIt.com

Stephenson, Joan. 2011. "City Living May Shape How the Brain Processes Stress." Journal of the American Medical Association

Stewart, William B. 2009. *Deep Medicine*. Oakland, Ca, New Harbinger Publications. Print.

"Stress in America: Our Health at Risk"; 2011. American Psychological Association. Report. PDF format. www.apa.org/news/press/releases/**stress**/2011/final-pdf

"Ten-year Incidence of Coronary Heart Disease in the Honolulu Heart Program: Relationship to Biologic and Lifestyle Characteristics.1983. From the American Journal of Epidemiology. Vol. 119, Issue 5.

Thoreau, Henry David. 1862. "Walking." First published. Atlantic Monthly.

Turok, Neil. 2012. *The Universe Within: From Quantum to Cosmos*. House of Anansi Press, Inc.

Veerman, J. L., et. Al. 2011. "Television viewing time and reduced life expectancy: a life table analysis." *British Journal of Sports Medicine*.

"Walk the Walk for Heart Health." 2012. Article. [Online] American Heart Association. http://www.heart.org/HEART-ORG/GettingHealthy/PhysicalActivity/Walk-the-Walk-for-Heart-Health_UCM_429892_Article.jsp

Walker, Evan Harris; 2000. *The Physics of Consciousness*. Perseus Publishing.

'Walking, A Step in the Right Direction.'2012. Weight-control Information Network. Article. [Online] http://win.niddk.nih.gov/publications/walking.htm

"Walking-A Whole Philosophy of Life."; 2012. Article. [Online] Walking.Org. http://www.walking.org/solemates-from-walking-org/solemates-walking/.

2008 Physical Activity Guidelines for Americans.2008. Department of Health and Human Services. ODPHP Publication No. U0036.

"6 in 10 Adults Now Get Physical Activity by Walking." 2012. Centers for Disease Control and Prevention. U.S. Government. Article.[Online]

"50Plus Fitness Waking." 2012.[Online] http://www.50plus-fitness-walking.com/benefits-of- walking.html